CU00932947

Nutrition and Diet Logic

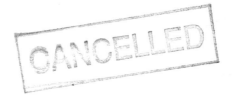

Nutrition and Diet Logic

Your Tailor-made Programme for a Longer, Healthier and Happier Life

Charla Devereux

foulsham
LONDON • NEW YORK • TORONTO • SYDNEY

foulsham
Yeovil Road, Slough, Berkshire, SL1 4JH

ISBN 0-572-01801-0

Phototypeset in Great Britain by Typesetting Solutions, Slough, Berks.
Printed in Great Britain by Cox & Wyman Ltd., Reading.

Acknowledgements

I would like to express appreciation to the following individuals and groups who have provided help and guidance during the preparation of this book: Deborah Beswick (Action for Research into Multiple Sclerosis), Dr Nadya Coates (Springhill Centre), Gillian Egan (Animal Aid), Joan Fisher, Charlotte Gerson (Gerson Institute), Tessa Glyn (Bristol Cancer Help Centre), Rayne Harvey (Environment for Hypersensitives), Rachel Holtom, Howard Hoptrough, Patrick Horsbrugh, Sally Hova, Martin Lev (ME Action Campaign), Trish Pfeiffer, Colin Ryder (New Approaches to Cancer), Cathy Savage and Gwen Vaughan (Living Earth).

Special thanks to Sally Crawford, who helped with the editing, and to Bill Anderton, the commissioning editor who made this book possible in the first place, and, of course, to my husband Paul who is always there for me.

Dedication

To my father who understood the value of proper nutrition.

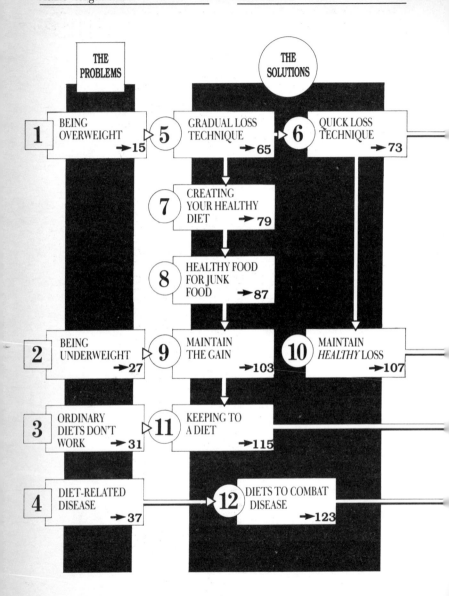

CONTENTS
CHART

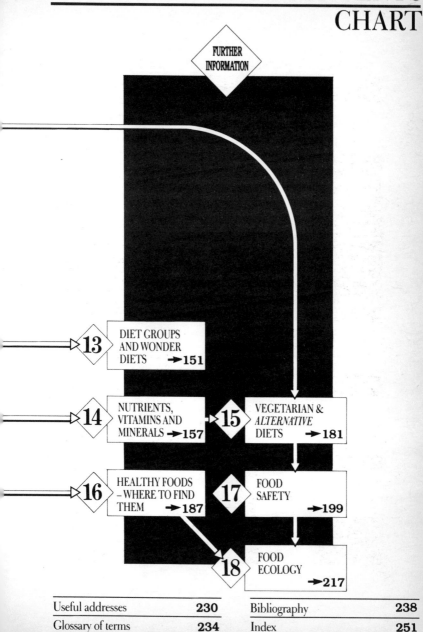

FURTHER
INFORMATION

Introduction

A number of basic factors, including diet, underlie the maintenance of health. Briefly put, these consist of having an adequate supply of pure water, breathing pure air and enjoying a lifestyle that allows us exercise, rest, emotional balance and peace of mind. The more closely we can come to ensuring a balance of all of these, the better we provide ourselves with the resources for a strong and healthy life. This book will touch on all of these essential factors, although its main purpose is to look closely at just one of them — the nutritional diet.

Whenever the word 'diet' is mentioned, most people conjure up images of half-filled plates of lettuce leaves and carrot sticks. The word is often associated with restriction and deprivation, especially in the minds of those who are continually 'going on a diet, starting tomorrow'.

There is an abundance of 'miracle diets' available, all of which guarantee weight loss if followed. The key to evaluating them is to ensure that they are *balanced*. A diet that is low in carbohydrates, for example, can reduce weight, but the weight loss will more likely be due to loss of fluids rather than a reduction of body fat. Furthermore, in such a diet valuable nutrients, especially minerals, may be lacking. The result is unlikely to be the increased vitality, energy and fitness that a balanced diet, designed to fit in with your particular lifestyle, *should* bring.

The actual dictionary definition of diet is, 'kind of food on which a person lives, a food regimen'. This book considers the many ramifications of this word 'diet': the importance of healthy eating, the connections with disease, weight loss, as well as the ecological implications — the 'politics of food'.

Before we explore the main 'problems' of the modern diet

and begin to come up with some 'solutions', let's look at your diet now. It is an interesting exercise to consider the value of each item of food eaten during the course of one day. What nutrients are provided, what do those nutrients do for your body, are there vital nutrients lacking from the food eaten that day? Are there any harmful ingredients? Bear in mind that any additives such as food colourings, preservatives, etc., need also to be considered. If your diet consists primarily of the same foods from day to day, this exercise may be invaluable.

It usually takes long hours of study and much practice to become proficient in any skill. Everyone wants to have a healthy body, yet its maintenance is also a skill. How many of us are proficient in that? Too often, the only sources of information available to us comes from what we read in magazines or obtain from radio and television. But how can we be sure that the information provided really has our best interest in mind – particularly in the case of manufacturers advertising their products?

It is perhaps hard to imagine a time before fast foods, a time when everything was made from natural ingredients right in the kitchen. Cooking was a skill that was learned and practised. To many of us today cooking simply means following the directions on a package of cook-chilled food obtained from the appropriate section of the supermarket. Most people feel that there are far better ways to spend time than shopping for the necessary ingredients required to prepare food from scratch, not to mention the preparation time itself! It is one thing to want to save time, but it is another to compromise our health in the process. In fact, as we shall see, it is perfectly possible to prepare healthy food quite quickly.

Many well informed people believe that diet has a direct relationship with disease and its cure or alleviation, and – better still – its prevention. The medical profession as well as those organisations who try to find cures for so many of the diseases that plague modern society should perhaps pay more *serious* attention to the role that diet might play both in the cure and prevention of those diseases. Surely it is at least possible that the quality, quantity and combination of foods consumed make some difference? Does it not appear to be the case that while Western society has overcome certain terrible diseases of the past, it tends to be replacing these with yet further scourges that in many instances can ultimately be traced to the kind of foods we nowadays consume?

The ways in which we prepare and grow our foodstuffs is surely relevant to health as well. Refined, processed food, as I hope to point out in later pages, can and does have an effect on our bodies over time that is analagous to the long-term effects of fertilisers and pesticides on soil. Dr William A. Albrecht, an American soil scientist (see *Secrets of the Soil*), has pointed out that preying insects and disease are not the *cause* of a failing crop, but the *symptoms*. These are all matters discussed elsewhere in this book.

The relationship of food to a healthy body and a healthy environment are not matters that can be treated separately. Now, more than ever, we need to consider the role of food as a single, powerful issue, relevant to the health of the body, ecology and economics as a whole. The purpose of this book is to gather these threads: rather than providing startling new research, it presents the key elements of existing information. Some of this information has been around for many years, and we can now begin to assemble it into a coherent framework of diet logic. In our culture we too readily leave things in a fragmented form so that the *whole* picture escapes our vision. This book is therefore a preliminary attempt to create an integrated picture of diet in a context in which healthy food is produced in ways that do not involve environmental damage, inefficient or unsustainable use of valuable, finite resources, and inhumanity – to our own kind or to any living creature.

NUTRITION AND DIET LOGIC

This book does not have a conventional 'beginning, middle and end': it is intended to be used more like a manual. (If you do read it from cover to cover you will find that there are a number of topics which are discussed in more than one section. This is because certain topics are relevant to different aspects of diet.) So to assist you in moving about within this 'new' framework of diet logic, the contents page is in the form of a chart. There is also a degree of cross-referencing within the text itself.

One final, important note. The term 'organic' is stressed throughout the book. While most people probably know the difference between organic and non-organic food, it is surprising just how many people seem not to. Indeed, there are those who actually believe that organic food means processed, 'new fangled' in some way, or, even worse, unhealthy! So, although there is a full discussion on organic food on page 222 and its accompanying table, it is probably wise to define the term here at the outset. The word *organic* is defined as 'being derived from living organisms and forming an integral element of a whole'. Concerning food specifically, it means that the food is produced using fertilisers that are solely of plant or animal origin without the aid of chemical fertilisers, pesticides and the like. In short, the way food was produced before the advent of modern agribusiness and the sometimes single-mindedness of excessive profit taking.

THE PROBLEMS

1 Being overweight

The human body is an amazing system of complex parts, each able to carry out its own function while working together to maintain the condition we know as life. Each of these parts makes many daily decisions — how the fuel (food) the body is provided with can best be utilised, for example. This decision-making is to some extent predetermined by evolutionary development, and although changes continue to occur, the timeframe over which these take place tends to be on a slower scale than the pace at which changes take place in our modern culture. This can lead to discrepancies between our preprogrammed automatic body processes and our 'modern' intellectual decision-making. Our modern tendency to accumulate fat is perhaps a case in point.

Have you ever wondered why it is that men tend to accumulate fat in the abdominal area while women are more likely to accumulate fat in the area of their hips and thighs? Recent research in the United States suggests that these traits stem from earlier times. Historically, men have been responsible for hunting and for protecting their territory. We now know that abdominal fat, the storage of which is promoted by an enzyme (lipoprotein lipase) found in the fat cells of the stomach area in men, responds to stress hormones produced by the adrenal glands. Adrenal hormones initiate the 'fight or flight' response and in these circumstances abdominal fat provided the required 'extra energy' needed for running, seeking prey or, when necessary, fighting. Women, on the other hand, have always needed a long-term energy store for pregnancy and nursing. Female hormones too stimulate the production of certain enzymes and these happen to be produced by the fat cells of the hip, thigh and breast, so that is where fat in the female body is stored. Women also needed extra long-term energy since they gathered most of the wild vegetables, roots, berries and herbs that provided the family with the bulk of their non-meat food supply.

Today's hunting and gathering is primarily done at the local supermarket; food preparation in many cases requires little effort other than buying and eating. In terms of effort, the average job too involves more mental than physical endeavour. However, the same biochemical processes take place in our bodies as occurred in those of our ancestors. Dietary fat is very easily converted into body fat and the tissue responsible for storing fat molecules can expand, almost indefinitely, to accommodate the excess. So what was advantageous for a society where food was not always readily available, particularly in winter if supplies were running low, is now detrimental in a society whose major food 'problem' is deciding what to choose. This situation is compounded by the fact that our diet probably contains a lot more fat than that of our ancestors.

The problem of being overweight, which means having an excessive amount of body fat, is one that confronts a large proportion of Western society. Excess fat can seriously affect certain body functions in addition to having negative indirect effects on a number of degenerative diseases (see Chapter 4). Many experts, as well as our own common sense, tells us that if we want to lose weight we must either *eat fewer* calories or *burn off more* of them through increased physical exercise. While this is true in theory, it is also important to understand what caused the excess weight in the first place so that steps can be taken to prevent it from recurring once the desired weight loss has been achieved.

Eating too much food is the obvious reason for being overweight. What needs to be determined is 'why'. If it is just a matter of not knowing how much food constitutes 'enough', or what foods are necessary to maintain a balanced diet that provides all the nutrients the body requires to function properly, then the rest of this book should provide the necessary information. A few simple adjustments to the concept of what you think a diet should be can dramatically increase your chances both of successfully losing excess pounds and at the same time attaining a healthier lifestyle.

Do not assume that because other members of your family, particularly your parents, are fat, that obesity is necessarily hereditary and that there is nothing you can do about it. It may well be that the reason fatness appears to be hereditary is due to a history of poor eating habits. If you were brought up on plenty of chips and other calorie- and fat-ridden foods, it is more than likely that these are the same foods you are eating now. There *is* something you can do about it. Blaming your parents is not the answer. Acting on the information available to them at the time, they probably thought they were providing you with a good diet. The trouble is, nutritional information was often minimal and provided by organisations that had more than a passing interest in promoting their products! Fortunately, today there are a number of organisations who are not connected to a particular product or industry but are dedicated to providing well-researched information about what is and what is not healthy and why (see Useful addresses).

For many people, however, the reasons behind over-eating go much deeper. It is important, as with any form of imbalance, to take steps to eliminate the cause, otherwise no matter how appropriate the cure, the situation is more than likely to recur. Of course, in order to eliminate the cause, you must first determine what it is.

A possible clue to what causes overweight can actually be found in the real reason why you want to lose weight. Although health is often a factor here, the real motivation may have something to do with self image, sexuality, or a sense of emotional emptiness; in these cases, the food may act as a substitute filler. Unfortunately, alongside the motivation, and more often mixed in with it, there can be guilt, depression, inability to make choices, and even fear.

So-called comfort eating is an automatic response that can occur whenever you are bored or depressed. It stems from being given a particular food (most often sweets) as a child, as either a reward or a consolation for any number of situations. However, once recognised for what it is, this Pavlovian type of response can be corrected.

THE GUILT THAT MAKES US EAT

If we can deal with guilt constructively as and when it crops up (as it is bound to from time to time), we can actually change it into satisfaction. A guilty reaction, for example, is likely to occur immediately if you see someone slip and fall on the pavement and you do not stop. If you decide to continue to your destination – perhaps you are already late – that feeling of guilt would probably continue for some time. However, if you went to the assistance of that person, the feeling of satisfaction that would bring, even if others had already arrived and the situation was under control, would more than make up for being a few minutes late. Long-term guilt may be a bit more difficult to handle but it too can ultimately be changed into satisfaction. First, though, it is necessary to determine where the basis for it lies.

Guilt usually stems from a sense of inadequacy; a poor self image. The roots of guilt can stretch all the way back to early childhood and can be so deeply embedded that only careful digging will enable them to be revealed. This can usually best be done by working with a qualified therapist. If you cannot honestly answer 'good' to the question, 'how do you feel about yourself?', then it is time to find out why. Overeating can be a form of self-inflicted punishment!

Trying to deal with the guilt arising from a poor self image, coupled with actual fear of being slim, causes a double bind, particularly since the fear is usually deeply hidden. Being overweight can in fact provide a web of security. It may act as a form of protection – by masking sexuality, for example. The cause may be that sense of inadequacy rearing its ugly head again, combined with a real fear of being sexually attractive. It is not uncommon to feel that you simply could not cope with either a sense of standoffishness from your friends or more attention from the opposite sex. Any weight reducing plan which alters your shape and clothing size ultimately alters more than just your weight; the way in which others regard you, and indeed the way you regard yourself, can all be significantly changed.

In spite of your best intentions, you can end up feeling 'safer' being fat and hating yourself for it at the same time. What first needs to change is the way you perceive yourself. This may well require outside help. Overwhelming guilt feelings can also be a symptom of depression. There are two main types: reactive and endogenous depression. Reactive depression is usually triggered by a particular situation, perhaps a change in circumstances or even something someone may have said. It is more difficult to determine the cause of endogenous depression, depression that seems to have no specific cause. Like guilt, the cause can stem from childhood. People who are prone to extreme mood swings or have a pessimistic outlook tend to be candidates for depression. It is always best to seek help in dealing with either kind of depression whether or not the source of it is known.

MAKING WISE CHOICES FOR OURSELVES

How we make our choices in life can have a major effect on how we deal with our depression, fears and anxieties.

Someone who has a problem – being overweight, for example, which is our particular concern here – will often proclaim that they have no control over it. It is always easier to put the blame somewhere 'out there' rather than take responsibility, especially when things seem to have become thoroughly out of control. The first step is to realise that, ultimately, *we all make our own choices* – even the choice to put the blame somewhere else.

Taking direct control over your own decision-making, especially to begin with, can feel strange, if not frightening. The initial decision is the easy part – in this case you want to lose weight. It is likely that this is not the first time you have considered making this decision but have been deterred by thoughts of sacrifice and deprivation. Even if you have attempted to lose weight in the past, one of two things probably happened. If you were unsuccessful in your weight loss attempt you may very well now make the decision that it is not worth trying again. By choosing to immediately accept defeat you are, in effect, reconfirming the belief that you have no control. If, however, you did indeed lose weight as a result of the technique you used, you will more than likely decide to repeat the experience, although you put the previously lost weight back on again. Your decision is thus a reaction based on past experience. By relying completely on past experience you may very well be destined to simply repeat the whole cycle.

Decision-making that relies on action rather than reaction can make the difference between creating a new reality, and thus a new you, or simply participating in another repeat performance. This makes sense when you remember that reactions are caused by past circumstance while actions have to do with current situations.

Now that you have made the decision to lose weight, what happens next? In order to keep the action from becoming a reaction (i.e. immediately joining yet another slimming club or going on yet another 'crash' diet) let us try another approach. It should be remembered that decision-making is a continuing process; it does not stop with one choice. In order to achieve the result of our intention it is often necessary to make regular adjustments to our actions. Choices come in different sizes. Deciding to lose weight is a big choice, but it takes a lot of little choices to achieve the goal. Gathering as much available information as you can about something always leads to better decision-making. The sections of the book that follow provide information concerning a number of aspects of diet, all of which you should at least be aware of. They will help you make choices that can lead you to achieve and maintain your goal.

First, two simple guidelines: try not to punish yourself (or, worse, give up) because some of the little choices that you may make turn out to be counterproductive. It should go without saying that we all make mistakes, for whatever reason. The important thing is not to decide to give up because of them. The only place to start is where you currently are. The second guideline is to remember to be kind to yourself.

The task of having 10 or more pounds to lose can be a self-defeating thought before you even start. No matter how many pounds you may need to shed in order to reach your desired weight, try to take it in stages. Make little goals for yourself, say five pounds at a time. When you lose five pounds give yourself some small reward — though make sure it is not in food form! The goals that you set for yourself should be in terms of weight, not time. Allow yourself all the time you need, you are worth it.

In summary, making choices that count is best done by:
- taking responsibility;
- acting rather than reacting;
- setting a series of small goals that are weight-related rather than time-related;
- rewarding yourself when a goal is achieved.

THE STRESS FACTOR

One of the most difficult words in the language to define is 'stress'. It can mean many different things to many different people, each equally valid. Indeed there are do-it-yourself charts which give a list of life situations and the amount of stress they produce. The items on the chart are usually listed in descending order starting with the most stressful. A value is given next to each item and the idea is to add up all the numbers which correspond to the situations in your life. The total is supposed to indicate the degree of stress that you are currently under. The problem with this kind of a chart is that it represents what situations are stressful in the eyes of the person who invented it. A situation which is stressful to one person may have just the opposite effect for someone else, depending, of course, on circumstances. The common strand lies not so much in the causes of stress, but the results of it. A certain amount of stress is beneficial; it helps us to make decisions and take actions that are part of every day life. It is when the amount of stress gets out of hand that it becomes dangerous. Constant stress will bring about changes in the balance of hormones in the body.

Our bodies have built-in mechanisms to handle the minor stresses arising from day to day situations. The adrenal glands produce catecholamines, hormones that are called into action to provide the added resources necessary for immediate physical activity. However, prolonged periods of stress can cause exhaustion to the adrenal glands, thereby opening the way for disease to occur. There are probably as many possible bodily reactions to stress as there are causes. It is often the weakest part of the body that suffers.

It is essential, of course, to understand the causes so that it or they can be eliminated where possible or at least handled in a manner that is least harmful to the body. Basically anything that threatens the health of the body or has an adverse affect on it – such as an injury, disease or worry — is a form of stress. So in addition to physical trauma, which can be caused by accidents, toxins in the environment, food or even extreme temperature changes, situations causing strong emotional trauma such as family feuding, pressures at work, and financial problems are all potential causes of stress. In fact the list is probably endless. Links between mind and body have been an accepted fact for many years and diseases such as cancer are thought to be more likely to occur in people who are highly stressed. It is believed that the natural hormones released as a result of stress can, if continued over a period of time, undermine the immune system.

It is important to mention here that certain food additives can also stress the body and this may contribute to emotional imbalance. A potential vicious circle could be set up whereby food is taken to try to satisfy the imbalance. The food, however, could contain the same ingredient that contributed to the imbalance in the first place.

All causes and effects of stress should, of course, be dealt with, and if necessary professional help sought; our primary concern here, however, has to do with over-weight.

FOOD AS A STRESSOR

One very common effect of stress, whatever the cause, is over-eating, particularly those foods that are least beneficial to the body. The feeling of not being in control of a situation, whether it is lack of money to pay the bills, a loved one who refuses to talk to you, or a broken ankle, can lead a person straight to the kitchen for a box of biscuits or whatever else happens to be around. Usually before you allow yourself the chance to think it through the unnecessary calories are well on their way to being turned into fat. The irony is you may not even like that particular food or those particular biscuits to begin with, and anyway you really weren't hungry!

When you next find yourself in this type of situation, and before you reach for the biscuit tin, try sitting down, closing your eyes and taking 10 slow deep breaths. Then just think for a minute about how you feel, why you feel that way and if having a food binge is really going to solve the problem. If you must, then binge on a piece of fresh fruit or a few carrot sticks.

WHEN INSTINCT BECOMES ADDICTION

It is interesting to watch how animals deal with illness. Very often they simply refuse to eat. On other occasions they may be found munching on grass and leaves in the garden or from house plants if they do not have immediate access to the outdoors.

Pregnant women often have cravings for food or food combinations that are not part of their normal diet or are not usually considered to 'go well together'. An instinctive craving for a particular food is the body's way of saying that it is lacking in a certain nutrient. When these cravings occur it is best to satisfy them, unless, of course, the same craving occurs all the time, in which case it is more likely to be a form of addiction.

Most of us are familiar with the effects of alcohol addiction because they can be so obvious. Not so obvious is that sugar also has addictive qualities. You need only try to refrain from eating anything that contains sugar for a few days to realise this, though in itself this is no easy feat because there are very few products – even savoury ones – that do not contain added sugar. It is, however, relatively easy to tell the difference between a craving and an addiction. A craving does not occur very often, and once it has been satisfied it will not repeat itself. An addiction will repeat itself, so if you find that you are continually longing for something sweet learn to satisfy it with a piece of fruit.

Choosing the best diet for you and your family could be one of the most important choices you ever make. With a little knowledge and planning you can create a diet that will be both beneficial to your health and leave room for modification when calories need to be considered. It should thus help you to eliminate the need for special diets specifically designed for slimming. Too often these 'special diets' can actually be hazardous to your health if followed for too long a period of time or relied on too frequently. High protein diets, for example, were popular because of their weight losing capabilities. The reason is that protein, eaten separately, will cause an increase in metabolic rate, sometimes by as much as 30%. The higher the metabolic rate, the more calories are burnt off. Unfortunately, the sacrifice of complex carbohydrates and fats in favour of more protein can have an adverse effect on the body in health terms. By being familiar with the various food groups (Chapter 13) you will soon understand why.

Finally, there is no miracle ingredient that you can take to lose weight. An educated understanding of the food sources available and what they provide is essential, together with a basic understanding of what the body needs in order to function adequately, but together they are all you need.

▶ GO TO ▶   ● *Gradual loss technique, page 65.*
● *Quick loss technique, page 73.*

2 Being underweight

Being underweight is most often associated with illness or malnutrition. Underweight should not be confused with leanness as a general body type; what is important is that you are not lacking in stamina and that a healthy, balanced diet is part of the agenda (see Chapter 7).

When it is necessary to gain weight, however, this can be as difficult as it is to lose it. Although theoretically the same ground rule applies – the more calories you eat the more weight you gain – the underweight person may have just as much difficulty in eating more as the overweight person has in restraining themselves from over-indulgence.

There are a number of conditions, including stress and depression, which can cause either a loss of appetite or overeating. The effect of stress on food intake is dealt with in Chapter 1. Regardless of whether excessive stress causes over-or undereating, it is essential that the causes of the stress be determined and dealt with in either case.

A dependancy on stimulants such as alcohol and cigarettes can also contribute to poor appetite. Excessive smoking, for example, can dull the taste buds and vastly decrease the pleasure derived from food. Carlton Fredericks in his book *Psycho-Nutrition* claims that a deficiency in zinc can also cause a loss of taste and smell. Such a deficiency state, however, would be something best determined by a qualified therapist.

Of course, appetite stimulation is an individual matter; what appeals to one person might be repulsive to another. The important thing is to discover what appeals to *you*. Some people, for example, believe that the colour red stimulates the taste buds — eating from a red plate may be the answer.

NUTRITION AND DIET LOGIC

In order to stimulate the appetite, it is often best to eat small meals at more frequent intervals than the usual three meals a day, at least initially. Alternatively, if a three-meal-a-day routine is easier to cope with, you could simultaneously reduce and eventually eliminate some meals while eating more at others.

Liquids should not be taken during or directly before a meal since this can contribute to a sense of fullness and cause a reduction in the actual food consumed. Drinking before or during a meal is not recommended in any case because it can have a negative effect on the absorption of nutrients, literally watering them down.

Anorexia nervosa is a more serious condition than simple underweight. Here a person, usually a young girl, becomes increasingly thinner because of complete loss of appetite. The condition is precipitated by a refusal to eat — ostensibly in order to avoid becoming obese. Most doctors agree that the cause here is psychological and usually the result of an overriding desire to lose weight; there is often a hidden agenda, however, such as not wanting to lose the sense of security that childhood can hold. A difficult mother/daughter relationship may be at the heart of the problem.

One sign of anorexia nervosa may be erosion of the enamel of the back teeth; this is caused by excessive vomiting, a common practice of those suffering from this problem. Often the person will eat a normal meal, or in some cases binge excessively on a particular food or foods, and then soon after, expel the food from the body by inducing vomiting. Whether this is done to give the illusion that all is normal to family and friends, or because the person actually craves the food, the result is the same. The food is eaten to gain satisfaction on some level – either for themselves or someone else, usually a parent – and then expelled before it can be assimilated by the body. Other signs of anorexia nervosa include swollen neck, broken blood vessels in the face, extreme weakness and, of course, underweight.

Whatever the cause or causes, this condition can lead to self-imposed starvation as well as hyperactivity. Laxative abuse can also occur, particularly when the person is 'forced' to eat. Laxatives are an irritant to the colon and when taken in excess can weaken its muscles; in addition, they deplete the body of potassium which can cause irregular heartbeat.

Anorexia nervosa is a very severe and serious affliction which requires professional help to both resolve the initial conflict and build up the body in order to prevent the inevitable outcome if it is not treated — starvation.

There are many factors, set up in childhood, which can lead, in later life, to poor appetite or unhealthy eating patterns. Teenagers are often influenced by fads and when it comes to food, nutrition is not usually too important a factor. At home children are often forced to eat foods that they dislike and so they vow never to eat them when they are old enough to make their own choices. These patterns often persist into adulthood. It is possible, however, to change these patterns as a result of new attitudes and values which come as a result of a better understanding of nutrition. By experimenting in the kitchen with the aid of a few good recipe books you may discover that the foods you thought you would never eat again are really rather delicious, depending on the way they are prepared and served. Clever use of herbs and spices can dramatically change the taste and thereby the appeal of many foods.

Living alone may be another contributor to poor appetite. For some reason people feel that it is not worth it to go to the trouble of cooking for just one. Why not? The complete answer to that question is something that could well be best explored with professional help. The common excuse that most recipes give quantities for at least two people should not make a difference. You can always invite a friend over for dinner. And for those meals when you do dine alone, you don't have to cut down on the amount cooked, the excess can be kept for another meal.

Chapter 9 offers additional advice for weight gain and this should be used in conjunction with the diet information provided in Chapter 7.

▶ GO TO ▶   ● *Maintain the gain, page 103.*

3 'Ordinary' diets don't work

Energy is essential for all living things. Plants utilise light energy which enables them to grow. As part of their growth process some of this energy is converted into sugars, starches, fats and proteins which in turn provide an energy source for animals, human and otherwise.

Energy is used by the body to produce the necessary amount of heat that will both maintain the temperature of the body and allow it to carry out all of its various functions. Our energy intake is measured in calories. While it is essential that we have enough calories to enable our body to operate optimally, the source of the calories must also be considered. Chapter 14 discusses in detail the various components of food and their relevance to a healthy diet.

It is ironic that most of us know very little about those aspects of health that are vital to our survival. We claim to be superior to animals because we are able to reason things out, but somehow reasoning often gets forgotten where things like nutrition are concerned. Animals know instinctively what is good for them. We humans tend to suppress our instincts and rely on what the experts say. We need, however, to first ask ourselves the question — what constitutes and in turn motivates an expert?

The closest thing to 'expert advice' on food that most people come in contact with is what they see on television or read in the newspapers, usually in the form of advertisements. Always question the expertise and motivation involved.

The amount of refined sugar we consume, for example, is of growing concern to most nutritionists and medical

practitioners. We need go no further than the nearest Wool-
worth's to see that it is big business — in some cases almost
half the floor space is given over to every kind of confectionery product imaginable. They all have one thing in common though — they are loaded with sugar. How many of the
people who eagerly purchase and consume these products,
often even prior to getting them home, have any idea of the
history of sugar and why it became so popular.

The sugar cane is native to tropical climates and was, for
a long time, nothing more than a luxury item enjoyed on
occasion by those who could afford the pleasure. Because
of its sweetness it was likened to honey and was sometimes
called 'honey without bees'. As early as 600 AD a process
was discovered which enabled the juice from the cane to be
refined into a solid form which did not require fermentation to preserve it. It thus became much easier to obtain. In
Islam, cuttings that had been taken as spoils of war were
planted and soon the eating of sugar cane became com-
monplace in Arab countries. The Crusades eventually
brought the Christians 'in on the act', particularly because
they saw the profit-potential of the crop. During the mid-
1400s cane plantations were set up in suitable terrain and
black slaves were brought in to cultivate the crops because
they were best acclimatised to the tropical conditions
required. By 1456 Portugal controlled the European sugar
trade, with Spain soon to follow. The Dutch established a
sugar refinery in Antwerp around 1500 and raw sugar was
shipped there for processing. Great profits were reaped
from the crop and the taxes that were imposed on it.

When the British gained control of the crop in the West
Indies from the Spanish, they turned the fermented raw
sugar cane juice into rum. This rum was brought to North
America and traded for furs from the Indians; the furs in
their turn were sold for high prices in Europe. Sugar
proved a very profitable industry, so much so that an objective of The Navigation Acts of 1660 was the prevention of

the transport of sugar from the American Colonies to any port that was not owned by Britain. In 1733 Britain imposed the Molasses Act which levied a hefty tax on sugar and molasses that did not come from British-owned sources.

When sugar was first introduced into Britain, sometime around the 1300s, it was a luxury that few could afford. By the mid-sixteenth century, the price had been halved and a century later Britain was importing 16 million pounds of sugar a year, the price being about a shilling per pound. The increase in consumption continued to escalate.

In 1812 Benjamin Delessert was awarded the Legion of Honour by Napoleon for his discovery of a way to produce sugar from beet. Before long sugar beets were planted throughout France and licenses were granted for the creation of sugar refineries.

There was much protest over the use of slaves in sugar production and finally in 1807 the French became the first to abolish the slave trade. It took Britain until 1833 to follow suit. Eventually the Americans created the ultimate in refined sugar – the pure white crystal variety. With nothing to stop them (the Pure Food and Drug Laws did not yet exist), and import duties reaping almost two cents a pound, America quickly became the leaders in the importation of raw sugar, a big business. (Readers who would like further details of the history of sugar are referred to William Dufty's excellent book, *Sugar Blues* – see Bibliography.)

Although the story of sugar refining explains why sugar is a common ingredient in a variety of food products, it does not explain why it may be harmful to health. For that understanding we need to take a brief look at body function. As part of the digestive process, enzymes reduce carbohydrates to simple sugars which can be utilised by the body. Once in the bloodstream, these are converted to glycogen in the liver and stored for future use, or converted to fat if the glycogen reserve is at capacity. The body uses simple sugars in the form of glucose, available to the cells through the blood circulation and as the glucose is used, it is replenished by the liver converting stored glycogen back into more glucose. Thus the blood glucose level is kept in a constant state of balance. About an hour after a meal containing carbohydrates the blood sugar level will rise, but only for a short period before balance is restored. Since it takes time for complex carbohydrates (the starches from grains, pulses and vegetables) to be broken down and absorbed, there is no sudden rise in the blood glucose level when these foods are eaten.

When refined sugar (sucrose) is eaten, on the other hand, it is quickly absorbed into the blood because sucrose is a simple combination of glucose and fructose requiring the body to do very little work to break it down. The consequent 'flood' of glucose destroys the balance and the adrenal glands are immediately called into action to produce the necessary hormones to restore blood sugar levels to normal.

Refined grain products are another area of concern as far as healthy eating is concerned. At least as far back as the medieval period, bread has been considered to be the staff of life. The grain used would vary from one location to another and while its quality sometimes depended on a family's financial situation, it always contained all of the nutrients that nature intended.

These days, in order to ensure a longer shelf life (which of course translates into higher profits) the grain used to produce the majority of the products on sale on the grocery shelves today has been devitalised through the removal of many of its naturally occurring nutrients. In some cases these products are then labelled with a term such as 'enriched' which, as the label goes on to explain, means that a proportion of these nutrients have been added back.

Since the body is *designed* to process whole foods it is

important that we *feed it* whole foods and let the body do the refining it needs to by providing it with all of the basic ingredients it requires to do the job.

▶ GO TO ▶   ● *Keeping to a diet, page 115.*

4 Diet-related disease

Thy food shall be thy cure — *Hippocrates*

Any study of the background surrounding the various diseases that most threaten our society (cancer, diabetes, hypoglycaemia, asthma, candida, arthritis, ME, etc.), throws up a number of common threads. More and more, such diseases appear to be a result of the evolution of our modern society.

Although it can be argued that the life expectancy of many of our ancestors was relatively short, the reasons for that had little to do with diet. Where death was due to illness, it was probably due to infections caused by factors such as poor sanitation. The main diseases that plagued the not-too-distant past generations (and continue to haunt some 'Third World' countries) included smallpox, tuberculosis, typhus, yellow fever and typhoid. Because of modern scientific understanding of bacteriology and virology, these diseases no longer pose a threat to our Western society. New diseases, however, have taken their place and it is important to ask ourselves why. To understand at least some of the causes we need to look at changes that we as a society have made.

There seems to be a correlation between adulterated food and many of the illnesses touched upon later in this chapter. 'Adulterated food' can be defined as any source of food produced by nature which has been interfered with by either the addition or deletion of ingredients, or any processed food made with or without natural, untampered-with ingredients.

There also appear to be connections between many of

the illnesses itemised below. For example, there are those who feel that hypoglycaemia is a forerunner of diabetes. When intestinal flora are destroyed and/or the immune system is suppressed as a result of large doses of anti-biotics, candida can often become a problem. As long ago as 1948 Dr Josef Issels wrote about the importance of the flora in the gastrointestinal tract being in balance. He felt that any imbalance where there was candida growth was one of the causes of cancer. For many years his writings were ignored by orthodox medicine.

Table 1: An outline of the immune system

The immune system acts as the body's main defence against disease and is responsible for identifying and neutralising foreign substances. It is made up of the following:

Thymus gland – produces a particular white blood cell (T lymphocytes) which help to resist infections including those from yeasts and viruses and protects against cancer and allergy development. The thymus gland releases hormones which regulate many of the functions of the immune system.

Lymphatic vessels and nodes – act as the waste disposal system for the body including drainage of waste from tissues and destruction of foreign particles. Certain white blood cells in this system (B lymphocytes) are able to initiate antibody production against invading germs when necessary.

Spleen – destroys worn-out blood cells and platelets.

White blood cells – destroy cells which are already cancerous or infected with viruses. These cells produce various compounds which aid in the destruction of the infected cells.

It now appears that any deterioration in the immune system (see Table 1) may be at the root of a number of modern diseases including cancer, skin infections, allergies, migraine, MS, psoriasis and arthritis. The body has a number of defence mechanisms which help to resist infection, each of which can be restricted as a result of inadequate nutrition. The outer layer of the skin (epidermis), for example, protects the body both from invasion by parasites and from becoming dehydrated. A lack of certain nutrients such as vitamins A or B-complex could lead to skin lesions which would leave the way open for bacteria to enter.

Nutritional deficiency does not have to be wide-scale as was once thought in order to have adverse effects on the immune system. Mounting evidence shows that even deficiency in a single nutrient can have a profound effect. Likewise there is evidence to support the theory that over-indulgence in certain foods, mainly refined carbohydrates, can significantly reduce immune system function.

There are a number of problems with the way orthodox medicine has developed that do not leave room for broader understanding. The most common problem is that orthodox medicine is geared to treat symptoms, usually by synthetic drugs, rather than to tackle the disease by the roots — in other words trying to understand what brought it about in the first place.

A fundamental problem with all drugs is that in addition to getting rid of the symptom(s) they are prescribed for, they can kill off many healthy cells as well, thus potentially producing one or more new problems. The spread of candida as a result of widespread use of antibiotics is a case in point.

Drugs are too often distributed without adequate testing. When I lived in New York, I remember one particular visit to my general allopathic physician which resulted in his giving me a few 'sample pills' that he had recently been given by a representative from one of the leading drug companies. At the time I was pleased about not having to take the extra time to go to the chemist in order to have a prescription made up, as well as not having to pay for it. Now, a bit older and wiser, I am appalled by such action. My doctor probably thought he was doing me a favour. After all, the drug company representative probably told him that the pills were thoroughly tested and perfectly safe.

I cannot help wondering whether the profit margin that good distribution of such drugs can produce is more of a motive behind the training and sales pitch of company representatives than actual knowledge of the benefits or testing methods of the product. I also wonder just how many drugs have been put on the market and then had to be withdrawn due to what was really a result of inadequate testing. Unfortunately, it is the patient who pays the penalty of an iatrogenic (treatment-induced) illness.

If an antibiotic is used often enough bacteria resistant to it can develop. Unfortunately, the usual response to this is to simply increase the dosage, or to try another antibiotic. As a consequence, new antibiotics have to be invented all the time – a process that cannot go on for ever.

The use of vaccines, often seen as a panacea, also have a fundamental problem. Any given vaccine is only good against one particular strain of a microbe which means that a flu vaccination received last year will more than likely not be effective against this year's variety. There is also a degree of concern that the use of too many vaccines may weaken or even damage the immune system.

Medicine has become a highly specialised field. The days of the 'family doctor' who knew everyone on a first name basis and who had a fairly thorough knowledge of the background of each patient are long gone. Different symptoms will be seen to by different 'specialists' and as a result any possible connections that might exist can be easily overlooked.

Our ultimate survival depends on the air we breathe and the water and food that we consume, yet the number of doctors who have little or no training in nutrition is staggering. Proper nutritional training should be a mandatory subject for all doctors and medical students.

With all the funds being poured into various research organisations it seems somewhat ironic that most of the diseases mentioned in this chapter are becoming more and more widespread. Perhaps more government-funded independent research programmes need to be set up to properly look into the connection between the foods we eat and the diseases so prevalent in our society today. Such organisations would have to be free from any connection with drug or food companies or any other group that could prejudice the testing criteria in any way. It may just be possible that with some fundamental adjustments to our diet we can curtail and indeed eventually eliminate some of these diseases. Twenty-six of the most prevalent are alphabetically listed below.

Acne
Acne is a common skin problem which usually occurs at puberty. It results from increases in certain hormones which then stimulate the sebaceous glands into producing excess sebum. At the same time an over-production of keratin (a fibrous protein found in the skin and hair) occurs. The excess sebum is blocked by the keratin and eventually blackheads or whiteheads are formed. Although acne usually disappears by adulthood, if it is not properly cared for, bacteria may cause inflammation to occur and this can result in severe scarring.

A high level of toxicity in the body may also bring on acne. The cause of toxicity can be from drugs, cosmetics, and exposure to industrial pollutants or household chemicals. A detoxification programme (see page 79) should be considered.

For dietary suggestions for acne, see Chapter 12.

Acquired immunodeficiency syndrome (AIDS)

The immune system is the defence system of the body. Antibodies and lymphocytes (white blood cells) are produced by the immune system to deal with damaging or potentially damaging substances. AIDS is characterised by the presence of the HIV virus and a dysfunctioning immune system where the necessary white blood cells are not produced in their required numbers and so the body is not adequately protected from infections and disease. Varying levels of severity are also a feature of AIDS, ranging from the asymptomatic state of no symptoms to the presence of life-endangering diseases brought about by severe immune dysfunction. There also seems to be a link between candida and/or herpes with AIDS since a large proportion of AIDS sufferers show signs of one or both of these diseases.

Although there is no known cure for AIDS at present, common sense should dictate that all known causes of immune system dysfunction should be eliminated while at the same time increasing all known forms of support. This should encompass stress factors, exercise, meditation and, of course, nutrition.

For dietary suggestions for AIDS, see Chapter 12.

Alzheimer's disease

This is a progressive form of dementia (a disorder of the mental processes) associated with degeneration of the brain caused by general destruction of nerve cells. This can happen at any age but is most prevalent in the elderly. Symptoms of dementia include short-term memory loss, vertigo, headache, ringing in the ears, depression, confusion and disorientation in time and space. It is important to note that although Alzheimer's Disease is considered to be incurable, other forms of dementia are reversible and a qualified therapist should be consulted.

Much has been written about the connection between Alzheimer's and the intake of high levels of aluminium over long periods of time. As food can absorb minute quantities of the utensil or container it is placed in, the use of aluminium for these purposes is questionable. Aluminium is particularly sensitive to acid and so highly acidic foods would be most at risk from absorbing aluminium traces. A survey published in the *Lancet* of April, 1989 showed that tap water boiled in an aluminium pot had 30 times the recommended limit of aluminium in it. It is therefore a wise idea from a health viewpoint to cook food in vessels made from glass, ceramic, stainless steel or, at least, enamelled metal.

For dietary suggestions for Alzheimer's Disease, see Chapter 12.

Arthritis

Arthritis involves the inflammation of one or more joints and is characterised by swelling, redness of the overlying skin, and soreness. A number of different types exist. Some manifestations are relatively mild and may only be brought on by wet weather or sometimes strenuous activity. This type of arthritis is frequently called rheumatism. Other forms of arthritis, however, can be crippling.

The two commonest forms of arthritis – osteoarthritis and rheumatoid arthritis – are discussed here. Osteoarthritis is a degenerative joint disease mostly affecting joints which bear pressure under weight. Maintaining a normal body weight and good posture are important in avoiding undue stress on the affected joints. Large bone spurs form in the joints as a result of destruction of cartilage (connective tissue between the bones of joints) resulting in a reduction of flexibility, deformity and possibly pain. Morning stiffness in the joints is characteristic of this condition.

Rheumatoid arthritis is a chronic inflammatory ailment which usually affects both sides of the body at the same time, affecting the hands, feet, arms, hips and legs most commonly. However, connective tissues throughout the body can also be affected. Immunisations – for example, rubella vaccination against German measles – are thought in some cases to actually cause arthritis. Another cause of rheumatoid arthritis has to do with dysfunction of the immune system where an imbalance in cell production can cause antibodies to be developed that attack the body's own joint tissues. Lastly, food allergy has also been associated with arthritis and may be linked with the immune system dysfunction often found in rheumatoid arthritis.

For dietary suggestions for osteo- and rheumatoid arthritis, see Chapter 12.

Asthma

Asthma is a condition characterised by abrupt attacks of bronchospasm, a narrowing of the air passages by muscular contraction, which causes difficulty in breathing. Major causes of asthma include allergy (from food or an external cause such as dust), infections, stress or over exertion. The best treatment is prevention and this involves finding the cause. In order to assess if the cause is food allergy, an elimination diet should be considered (see Food allergies below).

For dietary suggestions for asthma, see Chapter 12.

Atherosclerosis (heart attack/stroke)

Development of fatty plaque (usually cholesterol) on the inner walls of the arteries, can eventually restrict and even completely block the blood flow. If this happens in one of the two coronary arteries or their branches, a heart attack will result. If it should happen in an artery which serves the brain, the result will be a stroke.

Reduction of dietary cholesterol levels is considered to be the most important factor in the treatment of atherosclerosis. Many tests have shown that saturated fats play a key role in the formation of cholesterol (see Chapter 14). Indeed, societies where saturated fat comes low down on the menu have little or no history of atherosclerosis. Japan is an example of such a culture, prior that is to the introduction of Western culinary delights that derive from fast food restaurants. It is interesting to note that certain groups of people, for example the Seventh Day Adventists, have a low level of heart disease: it is surely not coincidence that they eat a vegetarian diet.

In his book *The 8-Week Cholesterol Cure,* Robert Kowalski claims that two further factors are important in addition to a modified diet. One is oat bran, because it has more soluble fibre than any other food source (as opposed to wheat bran which has a high content of insoluble fibre). This helps lower levels of LDL (low density lipoproteins) cholesterol levels. The other factor Kowalski recommends is niacin (vitamin B3), which is also thought to lower cholesterol levels. Kowalski points out that the connection between niacin and a reduction in cholesterol levels was first made in 1955 by Dr R Altschul. Kowalski also states 'Just why this information hasn't been widely disseminated by the medical community . . . I just don't know. But the facts are there, buried in dozens of rather obscure medical journals read by a handful of research scientists.'

For dietary suggestions for atherosclerosis, see Chapter 12.

Cancer

Cancer arises from the abnormal and uncontrolled division of cells that go on to invade and destroy surrounding tissues. This is usually due to a breakdown in the natural defence system of the body. Healthy cells reproduce replicas of themselves when necessary, but cancer cells reproduce abnormal cells, regardless of need.

In the 1920s, Dr Max Gerson, a German physician, applied diet therapy to cancer patients. This therapy was further developed in the 1930s and achieved very high recovery rates in terminally ill patients. However, a US Senate Bill to fund further research into Dr Gerson's therapy was turned down and he was suspended from his local medical society.

In his book, *Cancer as a Turning Point,* Dr LeShan discusses the use by cancer patients of meditation combined with a consideration of aspects of their lives they would want to change. His research showed that many of the patients he dealt with had experienced a loss of hope in their lives prior to their having developed cancer. The issue of the mind having an effect on the growth and development of cancer was a main topic of discussion at a cancer conference held in London in February 1990 which was attended by over 500 doctors and nurses.

The Royal Society of Medicine Family Medical Guide states that 'Chemical agents, inhaled or ingested, are believed to be the cause of 80% of human cancers'. In today's world it is probably virtually impossible for us not to be subject to at the very least inhalation of chemicals. A walk through any town, or any sprayed field, will expose us to any number of them. It is generally agreed that we all produce some cancer cells every day; normally, however, our immune system is able to defend us against such invasion. Problems arise when the immune system is not functioning properly. Indeed, many cancer patients are known to have impairment of their immune response.

In addition to known carcinogenic factors such as bad diet, industrial chemicals and high-frequency radiation, electro-magnetic fields are being looked at as another contributing factor. Not so much as a cause of cancer, but in terms of their ability to disturb the cancer cells once they already exist, causing greater proliferation. It is interesting, however, that for a number of years low-level magnetic fields have been used in hospitals in China, with varying degrees of success, to *treat* particular cancers. Perhaps it is as the medieval alchemist Paracelsus said: "The poison is the dose'.

For dietary suggestions for cancer, see Chapter 12.

Candida

Candida is a yeast-like fungus which occurs in moist areas of the body and is usually found in the digestive tract. Normally a balance is maintained between candida and friendly bacteria found in the body. The problem arises when there is a decrease in the number of intestinal flora (which inhibit the growth of candida) in the body, or a weakening of the immune system which controls the body's total response to disease. Either of these circumstances will cause candida to flourish.

A common cause for the increased growth of candida is the taking of broad-spectrum antibiotics. These drugs tend to destroy intestinal flora in addition to suppressing the immune system. Hormonal changes and pregnancy can also influence the spread of candida. The immune system may also be weakened by chemotherapy, steroids, environmental moulds and chemicals, insufficient nutrient intake, excess sugar consumption and excessive exposure to radiation.

Thrush is a form of candida which affects the mucous membranes or skin. It can occur in the mouth as membranous patches or in the vagina as a white discharge which can be accompanied by itching and soreness.

According to William G. Crook, MD in his book *The Yeast Connection*, yeast-connected illnesses are likely to occur in people who have taken antibiotics or birth control pills; they crave sweets and yeast-containing foods and beverages; they feel bad on damp days and in mouldy places; and they are bothered by chemical odours and tobacco smoke.

Until recently, there has been little to be found in the medical literature in Britain concerning candida. It has been suggested that because candida is not confined to a particular organ, it is not readily definable and because its discovery is still not accepted as medical orthodoxy it is simply overlooked. With the excellent work of Leon Chaitow and Gill Jacobs (see Bibliography), this situation will hopefully change.

For dietary suggestions for candida, see Chapter 12.

Cystitis

This is an inflammation of the urinary bladder, often caused by infection. Improper functioning of the immune system is another possible cause. There is usually a frequent urge to pass urine which then causes a burning sensation. Cramp-like pain in the lower abdomen together with the passing of blood in the urine can accompany more severe cases.

For dietary suggestions for cystitis, see Chapter 12.

Diabetes

Diabetes mellitus is a disorder of carbohydrate metabolism in which sugars in the blood are not properly oxidised to produce energy due to a lack of insulin, a hormone produced by the pancreas specifically for this purpose.

The symptoms of diabetes include an unquenchable thirst and excessive passage of urine. Women may also experience intense itching of the vulva. If severe, weight loss and abnormal tiredness will occur. Testing for diabetes is normally done through urine and blood analysis; however, a special glucose tolerance test can be done for borderline cases.

It is interesting to note that during the First World War the outbreak of diabetes dropped sharply amongst the general public, while at the same time it increased steadily amongst the armed forces. It is surely not coincidental that during the war sugar was rationed for everyone except the soldiers! They were given the sugar which the civilians had to do without, 'to keep up their energy'.

With the discovery in 1923 by the Canadian physician, Frederick Banting, of a method of extracting insulin hormone from animals, it became possible to keep diabetes under control.

Studies have shown that where sugar consumption increases dramatically so does the incidence of diabetes. A summary published in the *Encyclopaedia Britannica* in 1911 states, 'The excessive use of sugar as a food is usually considered one of the causes of the disease ...'. Banting himself stated that, 'In the heating and recrystallisation of the natural sugar cane, something is altered which leaves the refined products a dangerous foodstuff'. He felt that the way to prevent diabetes was to cut down on these dangerous products.

Although it is commonly known that people who suffer from diabetes must cut down dramatically on their sugar intake, adequate research has not been conducted to determine if sugar (particularly of the refined variety) is in fact the major cause of the condition in the first place. It was felt by British scientist T. L. Cleave in the early part of the twentieth century, that refined carbohydrates, such as white sugar and white flour, are harmful in a number of ways. Since refined products are more concentrated, it is easy to overdose on them. In addition, many of the valuable properties and nutrients, such as natural fibre and protein, are removed during the refinement process. The implications, however, of a massive reduction in the consumption of sugar would be enormous on the industry. The drug industry might have something to say as well, since insulin accounts for a good part of its revenue.

An article in the *Lancet* in January 1981 ('A high carbohydrate leguminous fibre diet improves all aspects of diabetic control') stated that 'These results, in conjunction with those from our previous studies, show that high carbohydrate, high fibre diets give appreciably better overall control to both non insulin-dependent and insulin-dependent diabetics than does the standard low carbo-hydrate diet still in widespread use throughout the UK, this being independent of calorie intake'.

Considering all of the information available that suggests the potential problems associated with the consumption of sugar, one wonders why The British Diabetic Association or a similar body has not yet funded a research programme to impartially determine if indeed sugar is a possible cause of diabetes.

For dietary suggestions for diabetes, see Chapter 12.

Eczema

Eczema appears as an inflammation of the skin, mainly affecting the epidermis (outer layer of skin). The most common parts of the body affected are the face, wrists and insides of the elbows and knees. Eczema causes itching with a red rash which can be accompanied by small blisters that weep and become encrusted. Scaling, thickening or discolouration of the skin may occur. A family history of eczema and/or asthma is not unusual.

Eczema often starts in early childhood and is attributed to a flaw in the immune system. It now appears to have been established that certain foods may be implicated in causing eczema. The only adequate way of determining if food is a factor is by a process of elimination. This can be a tedious procedure and indeed should only be carried out under the guidance of a qualified nutritionist or therapist. It is important to maintain a proper balance of all the necessary nutrients and so adequate substitution of food sources will need to be made in order to compensate for the foods being eliminated, however temporary that situation may be.

Although many foods can trigger eczema, it seems that the most common offenders are cow's milk and eggs, although testing is often done for wheat products as well as foods that have been artificially coloured or preserved.

To treat the skin, creams and ointments are often

prescribed and these can clear up the condition. If the underlying cause is not determined, the condition will more than likely flare up again at some point after the prescription runs out. Other possible contributors to the condition include stress and an overload of toxins in the body (Chapter 7).

For dietary suggestions for eczema, see Chapter 12.

Food allergies

An allergy is a disorder where the body becomes hypersensitive to one or more particular antigens (allergens) which provoke characteristic symptoms whenever they are encountered. This may be by inhalation, ingestion, injection or in some cases by direct contact. Immune system dysfunction, possibly caused by incompletely digested proteins, is among the causes suggested.

An antigen can be anything that the body reacts to as being dangerous and the immune system will mount a defence against it via the bloodstream. Food allergies can also affect different tissues and organs. Thus diagnosis is not straightforward and this could be a reason why there is so little available medical information that is helpful to sufferers. The idea of food as a potential antigen, however, is not new. Indeed, Hippocrates recognised that milk could cause gastric upset. Milk is recognised as the most common food allergen, with eggs and wheat close behind.

A distinction is made between food allergy and food intolerance. According to the ME Action Campaign's *Allergy and Food Intolerance Factsheet,* 'a food *allergy* is an immediate reaction to a specific food whereas reactions to food that do not occur immediately are considered to be food *intolerances.*' It is for this reason that intolerance to food is sometimes known as a 'masked' food allergy. In some cases, foods that cause intolerance in certain individuals are even more difficult to identify because they can be triggered by foods that are eaten regularly.

Whether allergy or intolerance is the problem, it can be very difficult to interpret whether or not food is the cause. There are a number of symptoms that can indicate the presence of a food problem but because these symptoms are extremely varied, any clear-cut diagnosis is difficult. The degree of stress a person experiences can also play a part.

The idea of using an elimination diet to treat allergy came in 1926 from Albert Rowe. He believed that chronic ailments such as migraine and eczema could be caused by food allergy. By the process of eliminating certain foods from the diet and then reintroducing them one at a time, it is possible to determine if particular food(s) are responsible for a particular ailment. Although any food can be a potential allergen, there are certain foods – specifically milk, wheat and eggs – that are most often the cause of food allergy. Table 2 lists a number of the ailments that may be caused by food allergy. It is important that all potential foods are tested, especially those that are regularly eaten. If a particular food is an allergen, the reaction will usually be immediate as long as it has been eliminated from the diet for a sufficient period of time prior to being reintroduced. A minimum of four days is usually required.

Table 2: Diseases that may be associated with food allergy

Of the 26 diseases discussed in this book, the following 15 may be linked to food allergy.

Acne	Hypoglycaemia
Arthritis	IBS
Asthma	Kidney stones
Candida	ME
Cystitis	Migraine
Eczema	Psoriasis
Gallstones	Ulcers
Hypertension	

Although a particular food may be found to be an allergen, all aspects of the food source should be examined before jumping to the conclusion that it is the food itself that is causing the problem. The widespread use of artificial ingredients added to foods in order to prolong their 'shelf life' (see Chapter 17), or indeed, the chemicals used in farming or hormones used in animal feed in the case of meat, could well be the culprit.

The ever-increasing number of additives, chemicals, pesticides and other man-made 'helpers' available to food producers suggests that patients with specific chronic symptoms should have food intolerance/allergy tests. It is estimated that approximately one in 10 people, including children, suffer from some form of allergy. Subjecting oneself to allergy testing by means of an elimination diet could just possibly save years of unnecessary suffering from one of a number of ailments.

For dietary suggestions for food allergies, see Chapter 12.

Gallstones

Gallstones consist of a hard mass, usually composed of varying combinations of bile pigments, cholesterol, and calcium salts, which form in the gall bladder. They can form due to an alteration in the physical characteristics of bile so that cholesterol becomes less soluble (as a result of either an increase in cholesterol or decrease in bile acids, lecithin or water), or as a result of inflammation of the gall bladder.

It is widely believed that the main cause for the formation of gallstones is a diet low in fibre and high in refined foods and animal protein. Food allergies may also be a factor.

For dietary suggestions for gallstones, see Chapter 12.

Gout

This is due to a defect in uric acid metabolism causing an accumultion of uric acid crystals (uric acid and its salts) in the bloodstream and joints. The crystals may also be deposited in tendons, kidneys and other tissues. Very often the first joint of the big toe is the initial area of the body to be affected and intense pain in the joint is a symptom of the condition. The pain, however, is intermittent so that periods of relief between attacks are common. Kidney stones are also common amongst gout sufferers (see below).

For dietary suggestions for gout, see Chapter 12.

Haemorrhoids

This condition is also known as piles and is characterised by enlarged veins in the walls of the anus. This results from a weakness that is usually caused by prolonged constipation, although haemorrhoids can also be caused by prolonged diarrhoea. Symptoms include severe itching.

For dietary suggestions for haemorrhoids, see Chapter 12.

Hypertension (high blood pressure)

The term hypertension is used to describe a higher than normal blood pressure. In most cases the cause is not known, although some hypertension can be caused as a result of other diseases.

Blood pressure maintains the flow of blood to various parts of the body so if the pressure is high it can stress the heart and blood vessels in addition to causing damage to other organs. Such an increase in blood pressure can also heighten the risk of heart attack or stroke.

It is felt that most hypertension can be alleviated by proper diet and a reduction in stress-related life situations. In her book *Lower Your Blood Pressure in 4 Easy Stages*, Dr Caroline M. Shreeves clearly indicates that one of these stages is indeed eating a healthy, balanced diet.

For dietary suggestions for hypertension, see Chapter 12.

Hypoglycaemia

Hypoglycaemia is defined as a deficiency of glucose in the bloodstream. It can be caused by an overdose of insulin, as was discovered in 1924 by Dr Seale Harris at the University of Alabama. Dr Harris noticed that symptoms of insulin shock, which was associated with diabetics as a result of insulin overdoses, could occur in people who were neither diabetic nor taking insulin. These people were diagnosed as having low levels of glucose in their blood — in contrast to diabetics who have high levels.

The remedy for low blood glucose suggested by Dr Harris was to give up refined sugar, confectionery, coffee and soft drinks, the items that he felt caused the trouble in the first place since they place undue stress on the pancreas to produce more insulin. The logical treatment for hypoglycaemia had been to eat sugar to raise the blood sugar. If Dr Harris is correct then it could be reasoned that by continuing to eat sugar the situation is aggravated since the increased production of insulin in the pancreas eventually leads to a breakdown in insulin production, the major cause of diabetes.

There is a long list of suggested symptoms connected with hypoglycaemia and these include extreme energy lags, extreme mood swings, depression, hostility, melancholy, fearfulness, crying spells, sleepiness after meals, specific food cravings (usually for sugary foods), hypertension, dizzy spells, feeling faint, confusion and abnormal behaviour. It is surprising that in view of this long list of potential symptoms, testing for hypoglycaemia is not a standard diagnostic technique. If the effect of diet was better understood, testing for such possibilities as hypoglycaemia (along with food allergies, see above) would be standard procedure before other diseases were diagnosed, sometimes erroneously.

For dietary suggestions for hypoglycaemia, see Chapter 12.

Irritable bowel syndrome (IBS)

This is a common condition where recurrent abdominal pain combined with constipation and/or diarrhoea occur over a long period of time. Excessive production of mucus in the colon and flatulence or nausea may also occur. Symptoms are caused by abnormal muscular contraction in the colon (large intestine). Infection of the intestines and stress have both been suggested as underlying causes.

A potential connection between IBS and food allergy (see above) has been recognised since the early 1900s and indeed papers supporting this are sprinkled throughout the medical literature. In their leaflet *All about the Irritable Bowel Syndrome*, the British Digestive Foundation lists food allergy under the heading 'The Irritable Bowel Syndrome is Not'. However, they do go on to say, 'although some patients find they are intolerant of particular foods, *like* wheat or milk' [author's emphasis]. Since wheat or milk are found in so many food products, particularly those containing refined carbohydrates, it would seem that further research into the potential connection between IBS and food allergy would be an obvious step.

For dietary suggestions for irritable bowel syndrome, see Chapter 12.

Kidney stones

Kidney stones arise when there is a crystallisation of substances which have been brought to the kidney in the bloodstream. They form where there is insufficient kidney secretions which normally keep these substances fluid. The stones, once formed, block the urinary tract and this causes considerable pain.

Kidney stones are usually made up of calcium salts and uric acid. Many tests have indicated that excessive protein in the diet is a major factor contributing to the high levels of calcium and that this is responsible for a high percentage of the kidney stones that occur.

For dietary suggestions for kidney stones, see Chapter 12.

ME (myalgic encephalomyelitis)

This condition is also known as chronic fatigue syndrome and was not officially recognised until the 1980s. It was originally thought that it occurred as a result of viral infection. Since the first observations of ME took place as a result of an epidemic outbreak, it was initially assumed that it did not happen in individual cases.

In *ME: How to Live With It*, Ann Macintyre describes ME as follows:

• 'Gross abnormal muscle fatigue, which occurs after a relatively small effort and from which the patient may take days to recover – quite unlike any fatigue ever experienced.'

• 'A variety of neurological (encephalitic) symptoms, most prominent being loss of ability to concentrate, impaired memory and disturbances of sensation.'

• 'Unpredictable variation in severity of symptoms from week to week, day to day or even hour to hour.'

• 'A tendency for the disease to become chronic over many months or even years.'

Long-term use of drugs can cause problems with the immune system as well as being potentially toxic in itself. It is thought that a healthy immune system in normal circumstances, will curtail the development of ME. In addition, ME in itself may well compromise the immune system further, leaving the body vulnerable to additional diseases. Any enhancement of the immune system function, therefore, would seem to be of vital importance in increasing the body's resistance to this disease or any other.

There may also be a connection between ME and candida (page 47) and/or food allergy (page 51) above. For further information on ME see Useful addresses.

For dietary suggestions for ME, see Chapter 12.

Migraine

This is a recurring, throbbing headache that commonly affects one side of the head. Blurred vision or awareness of flickering bright lights may precede an attack, symptoms which clear as the migraine develops. Nausea, with or without vomiting, may also occur.

Stress is often associated with migraine sufferers and food allergy (see above) is considered to be a major cause of migraine. Relaxation/meditative techniques should be considered.

For dietary suggestions for migraine, see Chapter 12.

Multiple sclerosis (MS)

MS is a chronic disease of the nervous system that usually affects the young or middle-aged. Myelin is a complex 'insulating' material that covers nerve fibres in the brain and spinal cord. When myelin sheaths are damaged, this affects the function of the nerves involved and this causes a delay in the passage of nerve messages. MS is characterised by numbness, unsteady gait, impairment of speech, weakness and varying degrees of paralysis and can lead to blindness and total invalidity. The symptoms that manifest depend on the particular nerves that are affected.

Although, officially, there is no known cause or cure for MS, it is interesting to note that the highest rates of MS occur in the northern United States, Canada, Great Britain, Scandinavia, northern Europe, New Zealand and Tasmania. Consumption of animal products in these countries is high and it may well be that a connection exists here. Indeed, Dr Roy Swank of the University of Oregon tested the idea of a low fat, low protein diet by monitoring the progress of diagnosed MS patients given such a diet, at all stages of disease from early to advanced, over a period of

20 years. The results were staggering. Not only was the disease arrested in most of the patients but there was actual improvement. For further information on MS, see Useful addresses.

For dietary suggestions for MS, see Chapter 12.

Osteoporosis

Osteoporosis may be defined as a loss of bone tissue causing bones to become brittle and liable to fracture. Women, particularly after menopause, are most at risk partly because levels of oestrogen, the hormone that helps to protect bones, are reduced. The most common areas involved are the spine, hips, forearms and ribs.

Although lack of calcium and other minerals contribute to bone tissue loss, merely increasing calcium intake may not solve a calcium deficiency problem if the calcium is not being absorbed properly. It may well be that there is an accompanying deficiency in stomach acid and this prevents proper absorption. Calcium must be in a soluble and ionised state in order for it to be absorbed, and supplementation with an appropriate form of calcium such as calcium citrate could be appropriate. This, of course, should be done under medical supervision, especially since some calcium supplementation has been connected with an increase in kidney stones.

The body works on a priority system and so if a certain nutrient is not available in sufficient quantity to service all the parts which need it, the nutrient will be distributed to that part(s) with the most need. In the case of calcium the blood takes priority over the bones, and, if necessary, calcium will be taken from the bones to ensure that the blood has the required amount.

Research has also shown that osteoporosis can develop from too much protein intake. It is noteworthy that vegetarians and vegans rarely suffer from this disease. A diet high in protein on the other hand results in an increase in calcium loss in the urine. An imbalance in the intake of calcium and phosphates can also cause a decrease in calcium utilisation and a good ratio is two calcium to one phosphate (see Chapter 14). Both sugar and coffee have also been implicated in leaching calcium from the body. Indeed, the formation of kidney stones may in part be due to increased levels of calcium in the blood that is filtered through the kidneys; it has to go somewhere.

In his excellent book *Diet for a New America*, John Robbins (who, incidentally, was at one time one of the heirs to the ice cream chain, Baskin-Robbins) says, 'The US National Dairy Council has spent tens of millions of dollars to make us think that oesteoporosis can be prevented by drinking more milk and eating more dairy products. But the only research that even begins to suggest that the consumption of dairy products might be helpful has been paid for by the National Dairy Council itself.' They must not be familiar with the research which shows a connection between osteoporosis and excessive protein in the diet.

For dietary suggestions for osteoporosis, see Chapter 12.

Psoriasis

This is a common skin problem which occurs as a result of abnormally rapid skin cell replication that does not allow time for old cells to be shed. This results in itchy, scaly red patches which form primarily on wrists, elbows, forearms, knees, legs, and the scalp, although other body parts may be affected. Unlike eczema, which usually begins in infancy, psoriasis tends to start later, in childhood or adolescence. The condition is often hereditary and sometimes occurs in association with arthritis.

A number of reasons have been suggested for the defect in the skin cell division rate:

• incomplete protein digestion which can inhibit formation of certain compounds necessary for cell reproduction control;

• bowel toxins which can increase formation of certain compounds necessary for cell reproduction control. It is possible that candida overgrowth in the intestines may have this effect;

• abnormal liver function (inability of the liver to filter toxins so releasing them into the bloodstream);

• alcohol consumption (which increases toxin absorption).

For dietary suggestions for psoriasis, see Chapter 12.

Ulcers

An ulcer can be defined as a break in the skin or the mucous membrane lining the gastrointestinal tract which fails to heal and may be inflammatory. More loosely, the term 'ulcers' usually refers to an ulcerative disorder of the upper gastrointestinal tract. There are several specific types. A peptic ulcer can result from abnormally high levels of acid and pepsin (an enzyme in the stomach which aids digestion). A reduction in the normal protective mechanisms of the lining of the digestive tract can also be a cause.

Gastric ulcers occur in the stomach and are caused by the action of acid, pepsin and bile on the stomach lining. When the same problem occurs in the duodenum the ulcer is known as a duodenal ulcer.

The presence of an ulcer can usually be recognised by pain in the upper abdominal area not long after a meal or during the night. The intake of food may give temporary relief, but the pain will usually recur about an hour afterwards.

There is some evidence to suggest that food allergy (see above) may be a prime cause of peptic ulcers. It is also interesting to note that emotional repression and/or stress are characteristics often associated with people who have ulcers.

For dietary suggestions for ulcers, see Chapter 12.

Varicose veins

When defects in the wall of a vein cause it to become disten-
ded, lengthened, swollen and tortuous, the result is a
varicose vein. The legs are the most common site for
varicose veins to occur, often as a result of strain caused by
prolonged standing.

There seems to be a greater risk of varicose veins among
obese individuals. Decreased tissue tone and muscle mass,
often caused by lack of exercise, also helps to weaken the
vein walls. Pregnancy can also cause added pressure on the
legs and varicose veins can occur as a result.

For dietary suggestions on varicose veins, see Chapter 12.

▶ GO TO ▶   ● *Diets to combat disease, page 123.*

THE SOLUTIONS

5 Gradual loss technique

The most sensible way to lose weight, particularly if you have more than seven pounds to lose, is to do it gradually. The most common complaint among those that either attend a weight loss club, or try one of the many quick weight loss diets that surface from time to time, is that although they are able to shed weight, once they stop going to the club or go off the diet, their weight returns. Very often they actually end up gaining more weight than they took off! There are a number of reasons why this happens.

Deciding to lose weight is one thing, actually doing it is quite another. In preparing meals for friends, partner or family, the first hurdle is how supportive they will be. It does not help to have food items that are not part of the diet around to tempt you, especially the ones that you are most vulnerable to. This just leads to unnecessary stress and can easily put an end to the whole idea of dieting on one of those occasions when you find yourself alone in the house when no one is looking. Another related problem is having to prepare two different meals, one for others and your own. More temptation — surely just a little taste won't hurt ... The fact is that just a little bit on the rare occasion really will not hurt; it is the guilt that usually follows which can lead, if you are not careful, to a binge. Equally dangerous is the fact that it can get to be a habit and this *will* make a difference.

Many of the 'miracle' diets that appear from time to time and claim to be the answer to losing weight are geared to quick weight loss, whether they actually say so or not. Total calories allowed are usually around 1000-a-day or lower, and as discussed in Chapter 6, this low level of calories is not advisable unless just a few pounds need to come off. In addition, if a very low calorie diet is used for an extended period of time there is more chance of cheating. Even if will power wins out, strictly adhering to 1000 calories a day can be a very difficult task, whether you are devising your own menus or trying to follow pre-arranged meal plans. Calorie counting is not all that easy, and the more complex the food the more calculations you need to do. When using pre-packaged foods that have calorie information on their packaging, it is imperative that you scrutinise this closely, or you may find that what you thought was 350 calories for the entire contents (which you have already finished off), is only for 4 oz/100 g-worth and the package weighs 12 oz/325 g!

Most diets will have menu plans that tell you exactly what you can eat each day. They very often add, sometimes in small print, something like: 'in order to achieve the desired results you must stick to the plan'. This may seem easy at first, but, unless conditions are optimal, it might prove to be a problem in the long run. Problems in sticking to the letter of a diet can too easily result in your abandoning the idea of slimming completely – or, at least, until the next 'miracle diet' comes along. Optimal conditions for dieting include, ideally, having all meals at home. For many people this may be only rarely possible, so prepare your lunch in the morning (or dinner in the evening if you are on alternate shift) to bring to work. Otherwise it could be difficult if your diet requires a baked potato or grilled fish but that is not what is being served in the canteen that day and a calorie-equivalent dish is not available. Further optimal circumstances for dieting rely on there being no unexpected invitations to dinner elsewhere, being able to find everything that is required for the diet in the supermarket in the first place, as well as strictly adhering to it.

Although a quick weight loss diet will more than likely

bring results when adhered to, what happens when you go back to 'eating normally'? If you are like most people, the weight will start to return. At this point one of two things may happen. Weight will continue to increase and before you know it, you are back to where you started from, or even heavier. Realising that you are putting back the pounds, you may decide to go on the diet again, particularly if it was successful the first time. The danger here is that this may become a pattern and if the diet, like many, is not nutritionally balanced, you could be doing damage to your body. Malnutrition means more than not having enough to eat, it can also be caused by improper balance between what is actually eaten and what is needed to maintain a healthy body.

Another important aspect that needs to be understood is body metabolism. Basically, metabolism has to do with growth and maintenance of the body and is brought about by the continual chemical and physical changes that take place. The term 'basal metabolism' refers to the minimum amount of energy that the body requires for vital activities such as breathing, digestion and blood circulation. This rate can be expressed in terms of heat production or calories. Additional calories, above and beyond those required for basal metabolism, are burned by movement. It stands to reason, therefore, that the more moving around you do the more calories will be burned off. That is one of the reasons why exercise should be part of every slimming regime. There are side benefits to be gained as well. Exercising makes you feel more energetic. If, however, you are not used to doing a lot of exercise, it is best to start off slowly. It is important to remember that exercise need not be something that you do only once a week for 20 minutes as part of a class. Walking is an excellent form of exercise. Where possible always walk rather than drive. Try to incorporate a 15-minute walk each day, even if you have nowhere in particular to go. If you concentrate on how you walk you can increase the benefits derived. By using your thighs as well as your legs you can increase your stride while increasing the number of muscles necessary to do the job, eventually building up to a brisker pace. If you have stairs in your house increase the number of times you use them. Simply by exaggerating movement, by over-emphasised stretching when reaching for something, for example, you can start to awaken muscles you never realised you had.

The idea is to increase your metabolic rate and this can best be done through an increase in voluntary muscular activity. Exercise contributes to physical fitness and this encourages more activity because it makes you feel better. Ironically, a reduction in calories can have a lowering effect on the metabolic rate, which means that in addition to taking less calories you are also burning off less calories. An added importance of exercise when on a low calorie diet, therefore, is to help ensure that additional weight loss is not hampered by the reduction in the metabolic rate.

No matter how good your intentions may be, it is very difficult to sustain a crash diet for more than a few days or a week at best; there are also the health implications to consider. In terms of sustainability, *it makes more sense to lose weight slowly,* allowing your body to become accustomed to a new eating regime. You will be surprised how your tastes can change. For example, if you are used to having sugar in your tea or coffee, try using less and less until you can eventually eliminate it completely. After a time you may well find that you actually prefer the drink without the sugar. Indeed, the very smell of a sugared beverage can become nauseating after a time. By developing *new eating habits*, gradually, you will be able to keep the pounds from returning once they have been lost.

Joining a slimming club can be a help or a hindrance or maybe a bit of both. One of the most positive points in its favour is that you know that you are not alone in your desire to lose weight. This is particularly comforting if you live alone or have a family that is less than completely supportive. Most clubs have a system whereby goals are set so that you have something to work towards and in addition you are 'weighed in' at each meeting (usually weekly) to keep track of your progress. One of the incentives to lose weight is to ensure that you avoid being embarrassed at weigh-in time because you may have put on weight rather than lost any. Even if you maintain the same weight from one week to the next you can easily feel that no progress has been made.

The best method for keeping track of weight is to weigh yourself once a week only, without clothes and preferably at the same time each week. If you belong to a club then it is best not to weigh yourself at home at all. You should, however, try to wear the same clothing each week since you will not be required to take your clothes off and different garments can make slight weight differences.

It is important to remember that there are a number of reasons why a slight weight gain – or no appreciable weight loss – can occur, even though you know you really tried during the week. One is the female monthly cycle and this certainly plays its part in varying body weight. Or, again, the effects of overeating one day will not necessarily show up on the scale the next. So just because you did not even come close to your allowed calorie intake on the day of, or the day before, your club meeting does not mean that you will have lost weight. It will also depend on what you had to eat the other five or six days of that week. There is just no getting around it.

Most slimming clubs offer guidelines that indicate what you can and cannot eat. Unfortunately, these guidelines are geared to weight loss and so little if any emphasis is placed on health, especially when they have their own products to push. Once you lose the weight, you are still faced with the situation of what will happen when you return to your normal eating habits. Chapters 7 and 10 offer enough information for you to be able to design your own eating regime and this will allow you to lose weight by actually changing your normal eating habits rather than having a special diet for a specific period of time.

If you do decide to join a club (see Chapter 13 for further information), or already belong to one, it really is important that if at all possible you do not miss any of the meetings. It is all too easy to feel just too tired to go, especially if you know you have put weight on. This really defeats the purpose and can lead to dropping out altogether. Excuses are easy to come by; weight loss takes time and effort.

Whether you prefer being part of a group of people with a common goal or doing it on your own, ultimately there are only two ways to lose weight and both involve calories. One is to reduce calorie intake and the other is to increase physical exercise so that more calories are burned off. As is true with most things, the best answer lies somewhere in the middle.

You may even decide that a health club which offers exercise facilities, or a weekly exercise class, would be better suited to you. These type of classes are available in most areas and usually cater for beginners. Although health clubs are more expensive, they may offer specialised exercise programmes designed to meet individual requirements and if you can afford to join, it is worth checking into. Of course exercise tapes and books are available for home use — although it is a good idea to attend a class for a while to get you going, especially if you have never done this kind of exercising before. Doing too much too quickly can be dangerous. It is also important to do warm-up exercises before getting into the more strenuous ones. This is true whether you have never exercised before or do so every day. Never push yourself to do more exercise than feels comfortable. A good rule is to do a particular exercise until you start to feel a slight muscular 'pull' and then stop, even if it means you only do three leg lifts and everyone else in the class can do 20. It only means that they have been at it longer. Each time you do a session you will find that you can do more and more. Of course, if you have a chronic disease or are extremely overweight it is important that you first consult with a doctor or therapist before joining a class.

Regardless of what method of slimming you decide is best, you owe it to yourself as well as your loved ones to be aware of the profound implications that surround the choices you make regarding the food that you eat.

▶ GO TO ▶   ● *Quick loss technique, page 73.*
● *Creating your healthy diet, page 79.*

6 Quick loss technique

Whether you have always been overweight or whether it is a relatively new situation, the process of losing weight can be an extremely frustrating experience. The desire is to shed it all *now*. Sadly, it is often impatience which stops weight loss from actually happening.

It may seem that a weight gain of the sort that makes all of the clothes in your wardrobe seem too tight happened quickly, but that is hardly ever the case. It is equally unrealistic to expect that the weight gained will just melt away even though you have not had a piece of cake or a chocolate bar all week.

To ensure that the weight lost stays that way it is important that you lose it gradually, at a rate of about two pounds per week. Although a crash diet will more than likely achieve quicker results, as soon as normal eating habits are resumed the weight rushes back – and some additional pounds may creep in as well. In addition, if a crash diet is maintained for too long a period it leaves the door wide open for a variety of health problems. As an example, the liver may be unable to cope with the potential build up of toxins that can result from quick weight reduction (see Chapter 7). In the final analysis, if you want to achieve weight loss and maintain it, dietary habits need to be altered permanently.

However, the problem may be just the odd couple of pounds that you need to get off by next week, in which case a low calorie (1000 maximum) diet should do the trick. The important thing to realise is that this *should not* be used for much longer than about two weeks. The idea is to lose a few pounds (up to five for the average person) quickly. Too few calories over an extended period of time can create the risk of health problems, but at 1000 calories a day, in addition to losing weight, it is still possible to ensure an adequate supply of necessary nutrients. In many of the very low calorie diets available these tend to be lacking. The health risk in that situation occurs because many vitamins, minerals and other nutrients work together, so a lack of one often means a deficiency or inefficient use of several.

It is important to have three meals each day so that the desire to snack before a meal is minimised. Balance out the calorie allowances so that you have two relatively light meals which will allow the third to be bigger. A suggestion would be 250 calories for the two lighter meals and 500 for the bigger one. At which point during the day you have the largest meal should be determined by your own lifestyle. Ideally, the largest meal should be eaten at the time of day when you usually feel the most hungry. Most of us have a vulnerable point and by recognising it and compensating for it you are more likely to be able to keep to the diet.

You can, of course, use pre-packed meals where calorie information is already calculated. For meals you design yourself, however, it will be necessary to have a calorie guide so that you can keep track of your daily calories to ensure that you are not exceeding 1000 a day. These guides should be readily available from your local bookshop or library. Calorie counting can become difficult if you prepare a recipe that contains many different ingredients and then only eat a portion of it. It is best to keep it simple. For example, fresh fruits and vegetables are ideal, not only are their calories easy to calculate, but they are healthier as well.

An unlimited amount of water and herb tea (or ordinary tea or coffee if you must) is allowed with absolutely no added sugar and preferably no milk either. If the milk habit is just too entrenched, then the calories from one of the meals will need to be reduced and this means a smaller portion.

Some meal suggestions are listed below. With the use of a calorie guide you can mix food items from these meals and the list of low calorie vegetables that follows them to create your own meals. Where grilling and baking are suggested the food should be cooked without the use of butter or oil. Indeed, oil should only be used in those recipes that specifically require it. Butter is not to be used at all.

All of the meals listed below are for one serving but the quantities can easily be increased to feed as many as required. Whether you decide to follow the specific meal plans given here or design your own, it is recommended that you include at least one large, fresh, raw vegetable salad each day and include a large selection of vegetables from the list provided. A list of low calorie salad dressing ideas follows the menus.

Please note: T = tablespoon; t = teaspoon.

Light meal suggestions 1 *(250 calories or less):*

a) 1 oz/25 g muesli with 4 oz/100 g low fat yoghurt and 3 oz/75 g (approximately half a medium-sized) banana.

b) One size 3 egg poached, two slices of wholemeal bread with up to 2 t of low fat spread.

c) 8 oz/225 g mushrooms grilled (1 medium-sized mushroom equals approx. 1 oz/25g), one size 2 egg poached on one slice wholemeal bread containing 1 t low fat spread.
(Note: no fats are required when grilling mushrooms; a garlic clove can be diced and sprinkled in the mushrooms before grilling if desired.)

d) 5 fl oz/125 ml unsweetened fruit juice, two slices wholemeal bread with 2 t tahini or 4 t sugar-free jam (if four teaspoons is too much, all the better!).

Light meal suggestions 2 *(250 calories or less):*
a) 7 oz/200 g baked potato filled with 2 oz/50 g low fat plain yoghurt with a pinch of dillweed or oregano for flavour, cucumber salad with non-oil dressing (see below).

b) 4 oz/100 g brown rice (weight after cooking) with 1 grated carrot, 2 oz/50 g cabbage, 1 oz/25 g grated hard low fat cheese mixed with oil-free dressing (see below). An apple (may be baked with a pinch of cinnamon) for dessert.

c) Fresh-mixed vegetable salad (see vegetables listed below) with oil-free dressing (also below), five crispbreads with 1 oz/25 g hummus or ½ oz/13 g sesame spread.

d) Wholemeal pitta bread filled with 1 oz/25 g low fat quark (soft cheese) and sliced tomato, cucumber and lettuce.

e) 4 oz/100 g wholewheat pasta (cooked weight) with sauce made from small can of chopped tomatoes, 2 oz/50 g textured vegetable protein (TVP – see Chapter 6); onion, garlic, oregano and basil.

f) Cauliflower cheese made from as much cauliflower as desired topped with 8 oz/225 g low fat yoghurt mixed with 8 oz/225 g low fat cottage cheese, crushed garlic, dillweed and ground peppercorn. (Blanch the cauliflower by placing it in boiling water for approx. 10 minutes. Drain, place in casserole dish and cover with yoghurt/cheese mixture. Bake at 450°F (230°C, gas mark 8) for 10–15 minutes.

Larger meal suggestions *(approximately 500 calories):*
a) 2 oz/50 g brown rice (weight before cooking) with stir-fried fresh vegetables. (To prepare vegetables, cut up an assortment from the list below, heat 1 T olive oil in a wok or frying pan and add the vegetables, stirring constantly for two to three minutes. Crushed garlic, a dash of soy sauce and herbs can be added for flavour). 8 oz/225 g of carob soya dessert (see Chapter 16).

b) 4 oz/100 g grilled or baked chicken (without the skin; garlic and herbs can be added for flavouring), 4 oz/100 g brown rice (weight after cooking), salad made from one or more of lettuce, cucumber, grated carrot and celery with oil-free dressing (see below). Baked apple made with no more than 2 t of honey (a pinch of cinnamon and nutmeg for added flavour may be used).

c) 6 oz/150 g grilled fish (cod, hake, haddock, lemon sole or monkfish) or 5 oz/125 g halibut with 8 oz/225 g baked potato chips (see recipe, Chapter 5). Ketchup (preferably a sugar-free variety) or vinegar may be used sparingly plus raw vegetable salad (choose from the list below) with oil-free dressing.

d) 8 oz/225 g baked potato with chopped broccoli, mushrooms, leeks and 2 oz/50 g cooked black-eyed beans (weight prior to cooking) cooked in 4 oz/100 g tinned tomatoes, chopped, ½ T olive oil, garlic, and garam masala, salad of 2 oz/50 g grated carrot and 2 oz/50 g grated beetroot with non-oil dressing.

e) 4 oz/100 g brown rice (weight after cooking), 6 oz/150 g sliced tofu marinated in 1 T soy sauce, one medium-diced raw onion, 1 clove garlic, 1 t chopped ginger root and dash of apple cider vinegar. Sauté the tofu in 1 T olive oil for two minutes each side, add the marinade, cover and cook on low heat for 10–15 minutes. Tofu and sauce goes well over the rice. Serve with small lettuce and cucumber side salad with non-oil dressing.

f) Pressure cook or boil 8 oz/225 g each of potatoes and swede with 2 leeks and mash (do not include butter or milk); garlic and herbs may be added for flavouring. Serve with one 'vegeburger' and raw salad made from any of the vegetables listed. Use non-oil dressing.

NUTRITION AND DIET LOGIC

CHOICE OF VEGETABLE

An unlimited amount of the following fresh vegetables may be used: asparagus, celery, courgettes, Chinese lettuce, lettuce, endive, okra, parsley, pumpkin, turnip, cucumber, cress, watercress, cabbage, carrots, bean sprouts, alfalfa sprouts, Brussels sprouts, broccoli, runner beans, peppers, mushrooms, onions, leeks, swedes, spinach, tomatoes, radish, cauliflower, artichokes, aubergines, Jerusalem artichokes, marrow.

Note: Keep cut-up celery and carrot sticks on hand in case an uncontrollable urge to have something to eat between meals should manifest itself! As an alternative snack, one piece of fresh fruit can be included from the following list: apple, orange, pear, half a grapefruit, kiwi.

LOW CALORIE SALAD DRESSING

Oil-free dressing can be made from apple cider vinegar or freshly squeezed lemon juice and a mixture of herbs. There are many herbs and spices that can turn a bland meal into a tasty delight and at no cost as far as calories are concerned (see Chapter 11 for a list of herbs and spices that are best for various foods). A minced garlic clove adds zing to this dressing and a dash of tamari also goes well.

Low fat plain yoghurt is another good base for salad dressing. A variety of spices may be added, depending on taste. One favourite of mine is cumin and fenugreek (to taste) mixed with plain yoghurt.

▶ GO TO ▶   ● *Gradual loss technique, page 65.*
● *Maintain healthy loss, page 107.*
◆ *Vegetarian and 'alternative' diets, page 181.*

7 Creating your healthy diet

Although a diet consisting of highly nutritious foods, in itself, goes a long way in helping to rid the body of toxins, you may want to start yourself off with *a three-day fast*. Whether or not you decide to do this, it is important to be familiar with the principles of fasting and of detoxification in general.

DETOXIFICATION AND FASTING

A toxin can be considered as any substance which the body regards as a poison. Although additives found in many processed foods are a major cause of toxicity in the body, it is important to remember that they are only one source. Unfortunately, no matter how hard we try to avoid them, toxins can get into the body through the air we breathe, the food we eat, and even the water we drink. Other sources include drugs, excessive use of alcohol, cleaning agents and chemical compounds found both at home and in the work environment, deodorants, aerosol sprays of all descriptions, chemicals used in the dry-cleaning process, and the dozens of chemicals in cigarette smoke (and you don't even have to be a smoker!). Even if you follow a healthy diet, you are unlikely to escape all toxic inputs.

The liver is the major filter for the bloodstream and prevents toxins from reaching other vital body organs. Those toxins that cannot readily be neutralised and eliminated, usually due to liver function being overloaded, will be stored in what the liver considers to be the safest place — fat. The reason is two-fold: first, toxins are fat soluble, and secondly, fat is usually the least metabolically active tissue and this makes it the most obvious place in the body where toxins can be left without doing harm to vital organs. The more fat, the more storage room; this presents a fundamental problem for people wanting to lose weight because toxins are released when the fat is metabolised. The body may react by actually causing hunger sensations in its attempt to protect itself from the release of too much toxicity. It can therefore be seen that detoxification should be a regular part of a healthy lifestyle and play a role in any weight loss programme.

Eating a healthy diet is, of course, beneficial in itself, particularly one which is high in water-soluble fibre, found in vegetables (preferably organic), oats and oat bran, for example. This type of fibre is thought to bind to toxins in the gut, promoting their excretion. Remember also that raw foods contain the highest concentration of nutrients, particularly if they are organic. Finally, you should be drinking plenty of pure water; this might differ from the stuff coming out of your tap. (See Chapter 18 for advice on how to determine water quality.)

If you incorporate raw juices into your diet, this provides another way to help rid the body of toxin build-up. Juices made from fresh (ideally organic) whole fruits and vegetables contain the necessary ingredients which, in this form, are easy to assimilate. These include enzymes which are otherwise destroyed during the cooking process and which help to keep our bodies in optimal running condition.

Additional steps can be taken to help rid the body of any toxins that might have accumulated. A three-day fast, two to four times a year, is an ideal way to allow the body to overhaul itself. Longer fasts can be taken, but I would suggest that they be done under the guidance of a qualified therapist.

Fasting should be done during inactive periods to enable you to rest as much as possible so that the body functions can concentrate on healing processes. Ideally, the last meal of the day immediately preceding the fast should consist of fresh fruit or fresh fruit juice. During the fast, plenty of spring water should be taken (at least 3½ pints/2 litres daily). Unsweetened herbal tea can also be included. The use of any substance containing synthetic or other chemicals such as soaps, deodorants and sprays should be avoided. It is best to limit food consumption to fruit and fruit juices on the day following the fast. Raw vegetable salads can be introduced on the second day and a full healthy diet thereafter.

It is also a good idea to use 'detoxified' household products. This can best be done by choosing products that are labelled 'bio-degradable'. Try also to completely eliminate all forms of aerosol spray, which also contain environmental toxins.

Toxins can also spread throughout the body as a result of a poorly functioning colon. To maintain a healthy colon make sure you have a healthy diet, especially one that is high in water-soluble fibre and low in animal products. (For further information on colon care, see Useful addresses.)

DIET PLANNING

'Everyone is unique' is a statement that helps us to realise our importance and worth, for indeed each of us is different in many ways. To understand oneself and one's uniqueness can be a life-long quest. However, physically speaking, we all share to some extent certain fundamental features. One example of such a common thread is the need to sleep. The amount of sleep required can vary substantially from one person to the next, but the important point is that if we do not get the amount of sleep that we need, our bodies will certainly let us know in one or more of a number of ways.

NUTRITION AND DIET LOGIC

Brain functioning, for example, will not be optimal so the tendency to make mistakes will be heightened. Eventually, if inadequate sleep persists, the body will cause involuntary sleep in the form of dozing off when you are in the middle of doing something else, like driving a car. That is why signs are put up along motorways to remind the driver that 'Tiredness Can Kill – Take A Break'. Those signs apply to everyone.

Another common thread is that food is the fuel that keeps the body functioning. Although tolerance levels and preferences will differ from person to person, ultimately we all need to eat a certain amount of food each day, unless, of course, we are fasting. This food must contain the necessary ingredients that our bodies require, unique in some respects but common in most. As has been said, when sleep is required, the body will ultimately force us to obtain it. *With food, however, the choice is more of an intellectual decision* and based on our knowledge, education, attitudes and social conditioning. The body will shown deficiency signs, in the form of symptoms, which if not recognised can lead to ill health and one of a growing number of illnesses (see Chapter 4).

Many illnesses that are prevalent today appear to be unique to modern man. So what is the common denominator here? *Could the answer to that question have something to do with the very food that we eat?* Common sense would dictate that the first step which needs to be taken to test that theory would be to understand what the difference is between the food consumed by modern man and the food consumed by societies in the past. Many people would argue that our diet now is better than in the past, and that this is proved by the fact that, 'people live longer nowadays, don't they?' There are, however, hidden fallacies in this argument.

There are in fact two arguments expressed in this viewpoint which, although they may appear to be saying the same thing, are subtly different. Let us try to untangle them. Our hunter–gatherer ancestors ate the type of food which encompasses the ideas of what many alternative thinkers feel is 'real' food and what everyone should be eating. Some archaeological evidence shows that tooth decay did not seem to be a prevalent problem amongst these ancient peoples; furthermore, health status is reflected in the teeth and bones found as a result of these archaeological digs. As an example, in the seventeenth century, a Dr Toope in Wiltshire used to grind up the skeletal remains he found in the many Neolithic (5000-year-old) burial mounds in that county to make an elixir. He noted that the Neolithic teeth were 'extreme and wonderfully white, hard and sound. (No Tobaco taken in those dales)'. Commenting on this in his book *Prehistoric Avebury,* archaeologist Aubrey Burl agrees that this was typically 'a condition nearer to the state of Neolithic than Saxon teeth', and remarks that two leading nineteenth-century Wiltshire archaeologists, Hoare and Cunnington 'noticed how undecayed the teeth were in the excavations of prehistoric barrows . . . there was little sign of dental caries at West Kennet' (a well-known excavation site). There were, however, signs of tooth loss and abcesses, but such conditions are due to poor hygiene and trauma rather than poor diet. So here is an important distinction for us to make, that is, *the difference between degenerative disease and infectious disease.* Degenerate means having declined in nature, character, structure or function from a former state. So a degenerative disease depicts a disease which causes the body to decline from a healthier state of being, usually over a period of time. An infectious or communicable disease, on the other hand, is something that can be transmitted from one person to another. What gets transmitted are infectious micro-organisms such as viruses. Transmission occurs usually as a result of direct physical contact or by handling an object previously handled by an infected person. Protozoa or amoeba are single-celled microscopic animals, some of which are disease-creating parasites that cause illness when they get into the body. The understanding of the importance of sanitation has gone a long way to control and in many cases eliminate the conditions where these disease-causing parasites can thrive. This understanding was unknown to earlier man and was perhaps one of the fundamental causes of a shorter life span.

Modern technology and understanding have vastly reduced the spread of infectious diseases in Western societies. In the process, however, we may have created a much greater incidence of degenerative diseases — *and it is precisely this kind of disease which is the major cause of illness today.* Just as we now know that pathogenic micro-organisms cause infectious disease, it may well be that in the future we will find that certain foods are the main culprits in the onset of degenerative disease. This is at least a hypothesis and one that is in fundamental need of unbiased testing.

Now that many people live well into their 80s and 90s, this is used as an argument that the modern diet is better than in the past. In most cases these people do not have a diet that would be considered optimum by 'alternative health' proponents. But the flaw in this argument is obvious. These people would not have had pre-packaged and processed food, nor today's almost universal presence of chemical additives and pesticides, as part of their early, formative diet. So they had a better base to begin with — *indeed, one that has now become the 'alternative'.* Our bodies really are remarkable organisms; they do their best to cope with everything that is literally 'dished out' to them. People who are now enjoying a healthy old age were brought up in a healthier environment from the standpoint of available food. It is a misrepresentation of the facts to ignore this when claiming that today's foods, which are full of artificial chemicals or those that are synthetically derived, are somehow an improvement. The real test of the matter will be to see how well the bodies and minds of the current generation of children fare; they are, after all, the first to be completely brought up in our polluted environment and fed modern foods.

The best way we have of individually dealing with the problem of degenerative disease is to take a serious look at the food we consume. As they say in computer parlance: garbage in, garbage out. It is important to be able to make educated choices, and that means more than buying a product because it was advertised on television.

Several points need to be considered when creating a healthy, balanced diet. These can be summarised as follows:

• high in fibre;
• high in complex carbohydrates;
• low in fat;
• low in cholesterol.

For further information on the specific points made above, see Chapter 14.

▶ GO TO ▶   ◆ Nutrients, vitamins and minerals, page 157.

8 Healthy food for junk food

In maintaining a healthy diet and staying at your desired weight you should be aware of those foods that provide no or very little nutritional value. You should also try to avoid those foods that contain ingredients that are less than beneficial. In most cases substitutes can easily be found (Table 3). The pros and cons of one food versus another are also set out below.

COFFEE AND TEA VERSUS DECAFFEINATED COFFEE AND HERBAL TEA

Caffeine is a component of coffee, tea, cola drinks and cocoa. It has been shown to be a stimulant. It is also addictive, hence the craving for that first cup (or mug!) of coffee to get you going in the morning, and for more coffee, cola, chocolate or tea to keep you going at other points during the day. Caffeine promotes wakefulness and increased mental activity which may be desirable in itself, but the caffeine-induced increase only lasts for a short period of time, usually just prior to the next 'coffee break'. Because of its stimulating effect on the central nervous system, caffeine can produce an increase in heartrate. When taken to excess it has been shown to cause symptoms of irritability, nervousness and insomnia.

Excellent substitutes exist for all products which contain caffeine. Decaffeinated coffee, of course, is readily available

Table 3: Healthy food substitution

If you currently eat or drink:	Try substituting with:
Coffee or tea	Decaffeinated coffee or herbal tea
Sugar (this includes brown sugar)	Honey
Chocolate	Carob (see Chapter 16)
Croutons in salads	Sprouts (alfalfa, mung bean, etc.) (see Chapter 16)
Carbonated soft drinks	Raw fruit/vegetable juices
White flour, rice and other refined grains	Brown flour, rice, millet (or other whole grains)
Packaged refined cereals	Organic oatmeal, muesli
Saturated cooking oil	Olive oil
Battery hen eggs	Free range/organic eggs
Red meat	Free range/organic poultry, meat and fish
Canned/frozen vegetables	Fresh vegetables (including raw salads)
Canned/frozen fruit	Fresh fruit
Fried foods	Grilled, baked, steamed or stir fried

and most restaurants now offer it on their menus. It is important to remember that caffeine is a natural part of the coffee bean, and some processing must take place to remove it. It is best to look for water-processed decaffeinated coffee (a term you will see stated on the label), otherwise the solvents (methylene chloride being the most common) used in other forms of processing may be as harmful to the body as the caffeine itself. For further information on other coffee substitutes, see Chapter 16.

Although there are numerous decaffeinated soft drinks

available, the best thirst quencher of all is water, whether still or carbonated. Water is second only to oxygen as the most important requirement of the body, and so an ample supply should be taken each day.

Decaffeinated teas are now also available, but the process for extracting the caffeine is similar to that used for coffee, with the same solvents and carbon dioxide being used. A wide range of herbal teas is available, however, most of which contain no caffeine, to satisfy just about any taste.

SUGAR VERSUS HONEY

Sugar originates from cane or beet which has been refined to the point of there being nothing left of any nutritional value. Brown or 'raw' sugar is really white sugar to which a bit of molasses and some minerals have been added. The molasses gives it colour and flavour; the minerals allow the claim to be made that it is more nutritious. As in the case of white sugar, they consist basically of empty calories. Many doctors and nutritionists claim that sugar is a leading contributor to many of today's modern diseases (see Chapter 4).

Many foods contain natural sugar, and as part of the normal digestive process that sugar is taken from the food and utilised. Sugar in this form is a vital ingredient for proper functioning of the body. If a natural balanced diet is maintained (including plenty of fresh fruits and vegetables) all of the sugar that is required by the body will be found, quite naturally, in the food.

For those of us who like to supplement our diet with added sweetness, however, it would be wiser to use honey as the source for a number of reasons. (1) Honey is sweeter than sugar, so less will be needed and fewer calories will be consumed. For an average recipe a substitution of between a quarter and three-quarters less honey than the required amount of sugar can be used. If you know your recipe you could even cut this down to half since most recipes taste just as good with less sweetener anyway. (2) Honey contains between 20-30% minerals and vitamins. The darker the honey, the more of these nutrients are present. Ideally, if you buy your honey unheated and unfiltered, this will ensure the maximum amount of nutrients. (3) Bees are sensitive to pesticides and so they will avoid gathering nectar from polluted fields. Pollutants that do find their way into the honey are usually a result of chemicals used by the manufacturer to make the job of removing the honey from the hive faster and easier.

CARBONATED SOFT DRINKS VERSUS RAW FRUIT OR VEGETABLE JUICES

Cola is probably the most popular soft drink on the market. These drinks usually contain a combination of caffeine and sugar, both addictive in their own right. In the sugar-free, low-calorie variety of soft drinks the sugar has been substituted by an artificial sweetener, but even this hardly makes the liquid a desirable product to put into your body.

Fresh fruit or vegetable juices are another story. Aside from quenching the thirst, they are a veritable storehouse of nutrients, varying only on the fruit or vegetable used. Because the juice is made from raw natural produce, all of the enzymes, normally destroyed when heated, are left intact. In fact, all of the valuable elements that make up nature's produce are available and easy to digest.

Rather than drinking empty calories in the form of soft drinks, it makes far more sense to make raw fruit and vegetable juices part of the regular diet. There are many to choose from: if you are in a position to purchase a juicer then by far the best raw juices are the ones that you can make yourself. An excellent book to have on hand is Thorson's *The Complete Raw Juice Therapy* (see Bibliography).

When purchasing ready-made juices, be sure to read the ingredients panel to ensure that there are not too many added extras.

WHITE FLOUR, RICE, ETC. VERSUS BROWN FLOUR, RICE AND OTHER WHOLE GRAINS

Common sense would suggest that a food that is in its natural state will be less costly than one where time and resources have been used to process it in some way. So why is it that white processed rice (or white processed anything for that matter) is less expensive than its whole grain equivalent? The answer, of course, is that processed products have a longer shelf life than whole grain products. The problem is that much of the vitamins, minerals and other nutrients that are found in the natural whole grain are removed as a result of the 'refining' process. Unfortunately, it seems that a higher profit margin often wins out over nutritional value. As the end consumers, however, we really do have the ultimate choice — so why not insist on food being organically grown as well while we are at it? Whole grains such as barley, millet and buckwheat, as well as rice, can all add variety to the diet.

Some manufacturers think that by throwing in a few 'enrichments' they can get away with the processed white stuff. Indeed many people prove them right by buying it, apparently being taken in by the cleverly deceptive bit of wording on the package.

In addition to the vitamins, minerals and other trace nutrients that are lost in the refining process, the fibre (see Chapter 14) is also removed. Why deny yourself these valuable nutrients? By using stone-ground wholemeal bread, wholewheat or whole rye crackers or crispbreads, brown rice, wholemeal pasta and 100% stone-ground flour instead of their 'white', literally de-natured counterparts, you don't have to.

PACKAGED CEREALS VERSUS ORGANIC OATMEAL AND ORGANIC MUESLI

The problem with packaged cereal is that the grains used have been processed. In addition, most packaged cereals contain added sugar. In fact most cereals are either fortified with or have added to them all kinds of things like vitamins which the manufacturer then confirms are essential for health, in writing, right on the packet. How much better it would have been not to have removed them in the first place!

As a direct result of growing demand by the happily expanding population of well-informed customers, it is now possible to purchase organic grains. For muesli, it is necessary to read the label carefully to ensure that all of the ingredients are organic, not just the particular grains used; most mueslis, for example, also contain dried fruit pieces.

SATURATED COOKING FATS VERSUS OLIVE OIL

The virtues of polyunsaturated and monosaturated versus saturated oils are discussed elsewhere in this book (see Chapter 14).

For cooking purposes the best oil to use is olive oil as it does not oxidise and become rancid when heated. From a quality standpoint, cold pressed virgin olive oil is best: the term virgin simply means that it is from the first pressing.

Olive oil has a very distinctive flavour so although it makes a good salad oil you may prefer something a bit lighter in flavour. Cold pressed sunflower oil or linseed are good choices.

BATTERY EGGS VERSUS FREE RANGE ORGANIC EGGS

It stands to reason that the quality of the egg will have a lot to do with the health of the chicken from which it came. Likewise, the food that the chicken eats will play a major role in its health.

Most eggs come from battery hens, hens that are kept indoors in relatively confined space. The only light that battery hens see is the artificial light in the hen house, and this is very often manipulated to stay on for long periods so that the hens produce more eggs.

Free range hens have access to fields and will be able to eat a diet that is more natural for them to eat. Organic free range means that the food the chicken has access to is free from pesticides and other chemicals (note that 'free range' does not necessarily mean that it is organic).

In addition to protein, an egg contains almost all the vitamins and minerals necessary for maintaining good health, with the exception of vitamin C. To ensure that the eggs you eat really do contain all of the vitamins and minerals that should normally be present, organic free range eggs are the best choice.

Although we have control over the eggs we decide to purchase, we cannot be sure of the quality of the eggs that go into the various baked products and ready-made meals that we buy. If the eggs used are organic free range then the label will indicate this. Any manufacturer who uses organic free range eggs in his products would be doing so as a conscious act and would want to make sure that everyone knew about it. The same would be true even if the eggs were just free range. However, if the ingredients list simply says 'eggs', you can be pretty sure where they come from.

RED MEAT VERSUS FREE RANGE ORGANIC POULTRY AND MEAT

Meat has been a valuable food source for at least as far back as recorded history. Hunting was a natural part of human existence. The meat that was hunted by our ancestors, however, had far less fat content than the meat that is consumed today. The animals roamed free and ate off the land. Pesticides, chemicals and acid rain were unheard of. Every part of the animal was used. Killing an animal was a conscious act and many people had rituals that they would perform that were directly connected to the hunt. The meat, like all of the food that they ate, was a gift from the earth which they received with gratitude.

As we know only too well, the situation today is quite different. Chapter 18 discusses the ecological problems that arise from factory meat production as well as the health implications.

It is now believed that too much protein, like too much of anything, is not a good thing. One of the first things that a therapist (allopathic or alternative) will suggest to a patient who may be suffering from one of a variety of modern ailments (see Chapter 4) is to cut down on meat consumption. It is also often recommended that the meat that is consumed be as lean as possible, and that white meat is preferred to red meat.

Some farmers are now starting to provide their animals with a more natural lifestyle and so free range chickens are now fairly easy to come by. This, of course, has come about because there is a growing demand. With a little more consumer pressure other forms of free range meat will also become more readily obtainable, and while we are at it, it would not be a bad idea to press for organic feed and pesticide-free grazing land.

While it is true that the price of free range meats is higher than that of intensively farmed meat, (and the price of organic would be higher still), it is also true that meat does not have to be eaten in the quantities considered normal by modern society. Reducing the intake of meat to no more than three times a week would make up for any price difference. There are many alternative choices available to provide the necessary protein (see Chapter 16). What is important to most people, however, is how much better the quality of the meat that is eaten will be, and how much better it will taste, especially if it is organic as well!

All processed meats really should be avoided. They are frequently made from animal parts that could not be used for anything else but are still considered edible. As Gary and Steve Null stated in their book *How to Get Rid of the Poisons in Your Body,* 'Frankfurters and cold cuts – everything but the squeak'. They suggest that before you have your next slice, a tour through a slaughter house may be of interest.

Fish, especially the oily kind, is a good alternative to meat and ounce for ounce contains as much protein. Oily fish such as sardines, mackerel, salmon and herring contain Omega-3 fatty acids, essential fatty acids that are required by, but not produced by, the body.

CANNED/FROZEN VEGETABLES VERSUS RAW VEGETABLES

The less that is done to a food the more it will remain in its natural state. This is common sense really. Alas, it is not the kind of sense that interests the average manufacturer. Manufacturers tend to be more concerned with what they can do to ensure longer shelf life, hence larger profits. Therein lies the fundamental reason why the majority of the food we find on the grocery shelves is not in its natural state. While it stands to reason that we do not want to eat food that has gone off, how many of us really want to eat food that has been sprayed with pesticides and chemicals, or that has been bathed in formaldehyde prior to freezing to ensure that it remains firm? Food irradiation, too, has been added to the list (see Chapter 17). One of the things labelling on packages does not tell us is which vitamins, minerals and other essential nutrients have been leached out or affected by these processes. In Leslie and Susannah

Kenton's book *Raw Energy*, a diet based on 75% raw food is recommended.

Organically grown vegetables are becoming easier to find and some major supermarkets now have an organic section in their produce departments. These foods are grown without the use of artificial chemicals and pesticides. The irony is that they usually do not *look* as healthy as the chemical-laden variety! They do, however, contain much more flavour, aside from the important benefit of having most of the nutrients still intact. It is best to choose vegetables that are firm in texture and free from blemishes. It is also important to remember that food which has a high water content, including many vegetables and fruits, lose nutrients faster than foods with little or no water content. Thus dried beans can be stored for long periods of time without affecting the nutrients they provide. However, the longer fresh vegetables and fruit are kept, the fewer nutrients they provide.

Another important factor is how vegetables are best eaten. All cooking destroys a proportion of the vitamins and virtually all of the enzymes. Canned and frozen vegetables have already been cooked once so they start off with fewer nutrients than will be found in their fresh counterparts. Of course, the longer vegetables are cooked, the more of these nutrients will be destroyed. Cooking can also alter the nature of the protein, fat and fibre contained within some vegetables. These are all important reasons why it is a good idea to eat a certain amount of raw vegetables each day. This can best be done in the form of salads or juices. A salad need not be a dull lettuce and tomato mixture with a few pieces of cucumber thrown in. There are many vegetables that are extremely tasty when they are uncooked. Be adventurous and inventive!

Some raw vegetables also taste good shredded – mushrooms, radishes and courgettes, for example – and this offers another way of including them. If you use broccoli be sure to use the peeled stems. The soft interior has a unique taste and crunchy texture that goes well in salads.

Salad dressing need not be the same old oil and vinegar mixture. Rather than using one of the premixed varieties, however, you can create your own very easily. Start with a base of good quality apple cider vinegar and freshly squeezed lemon, then try a pinch of one or two herbs such as oregano, parsley, basil, dill or marjoram, depending on taste. I always include finely chopped raw garlic to a dressing. A dash of soy sauce and a bit of cayenne will give it a wonderfully sharp flavour. Squeezed lemon on its own or with a sprinkling of added herbs also makes a healthy, very low calorie dressing.

Certain vegetables such as potatoes and artichokes simply cannot be eaten raw. You can, by the way, add left-over potatoes to a fresh vegetable salad. Beans and pulses, particularly the dry varieties, also need to be cooked, but can be added to a salad once cooled.

For vegetables that require cooking, there are a number of methods you can choose:

Stir fried – vegetables need to be cut into small pieces, added to a hot, (olive) oiled wok and stirred for a few minutes. A combination of vegetables can be used.

Blanched – pour boiling hot water over the vegetables (works best if the vegetables are first cut up into even-sized pieces) and allow to sit for a few minutes.

Steamed – add two parts water to one part vegetable, bring the water to the boil, cover and remove from the heat; allow to sit for a few minutes, the length of time will depend on the vegetable. Artichokes, for example, will take longer than peas. Special steamers are also available and these fit inside a pot and keep the vegetables from direct contact with the water.

Baked – vegetables such as tomatoes or aubergines can be

baked and the method is particularly good for potatoes.

CANNED/FROZEN FRUIT VERSUS FRESH FRUIT

Many of the arguments for fresh versus canned/frozen vegetables also apply to fruit. These include the following:

• the less done to the product the better;

• processing allows for longer shelf life, hence higher profits for the producer/manufacturer, the real motivating factor;

• organic produce is becoming easier to find due to increasing consumer education and hence demand;

• organic fruit may not look as pretty but will taste better and contain more of the natural ingredients that nature intended.

For the most part, fruit is eaten raw, usually not often enough though. Fresh fruit makes a good mid-afternoon snack, a healthier choice than biscuits or cake.

Fruits are digested relatively quickly and, ideally, they should not be eaten in combination with other foods. Pineapple and papaya are two exceptions. Pineapple contains bromelain, an enzyme which aids the digestion of protein. Papaya also contains a protein-digesting enzyme, papain, which helps the digestion of wheat gluten. A fresh fruit salad makes a wonderful dessert: to avoid any digestive discomfort, it is best not to eat it immediately after a meal.

To keep fruit at its best, allow it to ripen before refrigerating. Bananas taste best and are easier to digest when specks of brown appear on the skin.

FRIED FOODS VERSUS GRILLED, BAKED, STEAMED OR STIR FRIED

Studies clearly link a high fat intake with degenerative diseases such as atherosclerosis (see Chapter 4). These studies all point to the conclusion that the amount of fat in the diet needs serious modification. Foods that are high in saturated fats, the biggest offenders, are meat, eggs and dairy products. However, although olive oil is mainly monosaturated and vegetable oils are mainly polyunsaturated, it should be remembered that they are still 100% fat.

Since there are a number of ways that food which requires cooking can be prepared, it is unnecessary to have to fry anything. The primary reason for not frying food is to avoid an obvious additional source of fat and calories.

There are additional reasons why it may be unwise to order fried food when eating outside the home. Firstly, it is unlikely that pure virgin olive oil will be used because of the high cost. Another reason is that oils tend to be reused a number of times, particularly in fast food restaurants, and this is not conducive to optimal health.

Since added fat is not required for grilled or baked foods, these methods make the best substitutes for frying, especially for fish or poultry. A number of vegetables such as mushrooms and peppers (particularly red peppers) are also very good grilled. Steaming is a good method of cooking vegetables, keeping in mind that the less time food is cooked the less nutritional loss will occur. A little oil is required for stir fried foods, but because the actual cooking time is fast, this method too is a better choice than traditional frying.

Even potato chips and other potato dishes can be made without frying. First, boil or pressure cook the potatoes. I recommend leaving the skin on, and, of course, using organic potatoes. Next, drain, slice, and place them on a baking sheet and bake for approximately 30 minutes in a

Table 4: Suggested snack foods (including calorie count) that make good substitutes for manufactured snacks

Single piece of fruit (unless otherwise stated)	Kcal	Crackers	
Apple	50	Light crispbread	20
Clementine	25	Rice cake	30
Date	15	Ryvita	26
Fig (fresh)	15	high fibre	23
Grapefruit (½)	25	sesame seed	31
Grape	5	Scoople	23
Kiwi	35		
Mandarin	20	Cracker toppings (per level teaspoon)	
Orange (small)	35	Jam (reduced sugar)	8
Pear	50	Vegetarian spread	
Pineapple ring	20	mushroom	16
Plum	10	herbs	13
Satsuma	20	olive	15
Strawberries (7 oz)	50	tomato	17
Tangerine	20	Marmite	9
		Cottage cheese	5
Vegetable		Pear and apple spread	12
Carrot (2 oz)	12	Edam	15
Celery stick	5	Dutch 12% fat	11
		Quark low-fat	6
		Cheddar reduced fat	14
		Cheshire reduced fat	13

Note: Allow no more than 50 calories per snack – once a day maximum.

preheated oven (375°F, 190°C, gas mark 5). Home fried without the frying!

OTHER CONSIDERATIONS

All junk foods should be eliminated from the diet. Under this heading come all processed products, especially those where you need the help of a chemical chart in order to identify the ingredients. Aside from lacking nutrients, junk foods can be addictive, not necessarily by accident. The added sugar (sucrose) found in some sweet foods (choco-late, cake, biscuits, etc.) causes a rapid increase in the blood sugar level, especially if they are eaten as a snack on an empty stomach. This gives the illusion of the food being good for you because of the sudden rush of energy. In its attempt to counteract the blood sugar imbalance, the body can cause it to drop just as quickly, sometimes to an abnormally low level. If another sugary piece of food is eaten, because of the sudden energy drain, the whole process starts all over again. Table 4 gives a list of suggested alternative snack foods and their calorie count.

Another ingredient commonly found in junk foods is salt. Excessive salt in the diet can lead to high blood pressure (see Chapter 17). Salt (sodium) occurs naturally in many foods and this actually makes it unnecessary to have to add it to food in order to meet body requirements.

As mentioned earlier, everyone is unique. Translated into diet terms this means that to a degree different people have different dietary requirements. Some people may require more calcium than others, for instance. It may be well worthwhile to visit a nutritional consultant, preferably one who is not trying to sell a particular product. They can analyse what condition your body is in and what nutrients may be lacking. A good therapist will recommend the best food choices for your particular needs. If a nutrient deficiency is determined a supplement could be recommended to help restore the imbalance.

Although many people take multivitamins regularly, these are probably not required if you are eating a healthy diet. They may, however, be advisable for those periods of time when deviation from your regular diet takes place. This may be as a result of reduced calories due to slimming, or when you are away from home and have less control over the foods you eat.

▶ GO TO ▶   ● *Maintain the gain, page 103.*
              ◆ *Nutrients, vitamins and minerals, page 157.*

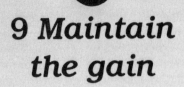

9 Maintain the gain

The idea of being able to eat all of those high calorie foods that are so delicious but are a major factor of obesity surely must be a slimmer's dream, at least initially. An educated slimmer really should know better. Believe it or not, where health is the main objective, it is more difficult to design a diet that is high in calorie-rich foods than one which is not.

The main aim in gaining weight, of course, is to consume more calories each day than are expended by the involuntary and voluntary processes of the body. It is probably a good strategy to have added snacks during the day – at midmorning, mid-afternoon and bedtime – especially if it is difficult to increase the amount of food consumed at mealtimes due to lack of appetite. It is also a good idea to have a variety of different foods at each meal. It has been shown that people who are restricted to one food will usually eat considerably less of it than if a choice of foods are available. An increase in the intake of concentrated complex carbohydrates (wholemeal bread, cereals and pasta) is also a good idea, particularly as such foods can be topped with extra calories in the form of various nut butters, jam (preferably sweetened with honey), and tomato sauce, for example.

A list of high calorie healthy food snack ideas along with a few other helpful hints are given below; all can be used to supplement the healthy diet discussed in Chapter 7.

FRUIT AND VEGETABLE SNACKS

Avocado pears – these contain 223 calories per 4 oz/100 g

(half a medium-sized avocado) and are high in protein, vitamin B-complex, vitamin E, minerals and polyunsaturated fats. Avocado can be eaten on its own or cut up in a salad. Rub the avocado with lemon juice to prevent it from turning brown. It also makes a good salad on its own with grated raw beetroot. Guacamole (avocado dip) is a delicious dip or pitta bread filler. It is simple to make; blend one avocado, 1 tablespoon fresh lemon juice, one crushed garlic clove, a dash of cayenne pepper and tamari or soy sauce to taste.

Cheese – grated hard cheese such as red Leicester or Cheddar can be used as a filling for one or two baked potatoes.

Creamy sauces – a tasty sauce can be made using melted cheese or cream as a base with a variety of spices for added flavour. This goes well on just about any steamed vegetable.

Dried fruit – although a dried apricot has the same number of calories as a fresh one (the difference being the water content which contains no calories), more than one at a time of the dried variety is usually eaten. Dried fruits can make a good snack. However, some manufacturers treat their products with sulphur dioxide or coat them with mineral oil. The better option is to buy the ones that are coated with a good quality vegetable oil, or not coated at all. It is also a good idea to avoid the added sulphur dioxide. Uncoated dried fruit containing no sulphur dioxide is available in most healthfood shops.

High calorie dressings – a sufficient quantity of raw vegetables is still advisable if you are on a weight gaining diet. Even though they do not provide an abundance of calories, the nutrients they do provide makes up for it. Olive oil (other recommended oils include linseed, sunflower and soya) should be used as part of the dressing and can be mixed with apple cider vinegar, wine vinegar or lemon juice and herbs. Shredded hard cheese gives a piquant flavour along with some added calories. Olives provide another tasty addition.

OTHER SNACKS

Tahini (see Chapter 16) – high in nutrients as well as calories. It makes a wonderful added ingredient in hummus. All you need to do is blend 1 cup (dry weight) cooked chickpeas, 3 garlic cloves, the juice of one freshly squeezed lemon, 2 tablespoons olive oil, 3 tablespoons apple cider vinegar, 6 oz/150 g minced onions and tahini (sesame paste) to taste. This goes well on pitta bread or crackers.

Cream cheese – because it contains more fat, cream cheese is higher in calories than most other cheeses. It can be used on crackers; try including some sliced banana for variation.

MAIN MEAL SUGGESTIONS

Nuts – these are another nutritional food source, as well as being relatively high in calories. Nut cutlets or loaves are common vegetarian dishes. There are a number of companies that provide pre-packaged nut-based dishes which are also full of other good ingredients (see Chapter 16).

Melted cheese – used as a topping, this tastes good on vegeburgers. Grated hard cheese also tastes good scrambled in with eggs.

High calorie sauces – these are a delicious way of providing a meal with added calories. Here are a couple of suggestions (T = tablespoon; t = teaspoon):

1. Peanut sauce is easy to make. Apart from providing additional calories, it makes a mouth-watering topping for chicken, tofu and all sorts of vegetables. Combine 2½ T crunchy peanut butter, ½ T tomato ketchup, 1 t sweet chilli sauce, 1 t minced ginger root, 1 t shredded coconut, 7 fl oz/ 200 ml sweetened soya milk and 2 t Worcestershire sauce. Slowly bring to the boil, stirring continuously. Peanut sauce can either be served immediately or allowed to cool.

2. Tomato sauce is also easy to prepare. Place 2 T olive oil in a pan with diced garlic and heat until garlic starts to sizzle. Add 1 can of peeled diced tomatoes along with basil and oregano to taste, together with a pinch of cayenne. Allow to simmer for about 15 minutes. Use over pasta, potatoes or vegetables. Parmesan cheese (or any hard cheese) can be grated over the top.

NOTE: An intake of excessively fatty foods is not to be encouraged for prolonged periods of time. For chronic weight gain problems a visit to a qualified nutritionist or therapist is essential.

▶ GO TO ▶   ◆ *Nutrients, vitamins and minerals, page 157.*

10 Maintain healthy loss

There is no getting around the fact that controlling calorie intake is the most effective way of controlling body weight. When contemplating a diet, many people never get beyond the thought that it might be necessary to dramatically alter their eating habits. Change does not come easily, especially when what may require elimination are the very things that we enjoy and look forward to. In order to ensure the desired results, in this case weight loss, every step should be taken gradually rather than trying to change what may be a lifetime of eating habits overnight (see Chapter 5).

Table 5: Food substitutions that help reduce calorie intake

If you currently use:	Try substituting with:
Whole milk	Skimmed milk
Butter or margarine	Low-fat spreads
Cheese	Low-fat cheese, cottage cheese
Fatty meats such as pork, duck, goose, sausage	Lean meat and poultry without the skin, fish
Chocolates, boiled sweets, other confectionery, crisps, etc. for between meal snacks	Fresh fruit
Chips	Baked potato or oven chipped
Fried foods	Baked, grilled or stir fried

When considering dietary changes for either weight loss or health reasons, it is worth trying first of all to substitute the more fattening foods in your diet with lower-calorie versions (see Table 5), rather than simply cutting items out altogether. Not only are the substituted foods likely to be healthier, it means you do not initially have to drastically alter your eating patterns. You can slowly modify your diet at the same time as you are losing weight, which will ultimately lead to a slimmer and healthier you — permanently.

LOW CALORIE SUBSTITUTIONS

Skimmed milk for whole milk

There are twice as many calories in silver top milk as there are in skimmed milk: per pint, silver top contains 380 calories; skimmed milk has 190 calories. So if you are one of those people who add milk to tea, coffee or breakfast cereals, switching to skimmed milk is a good place to start to trim calories. It is an even better start if you currently use cream, as one pint of single cream contains 1120 calories. Even higher are imitation and non-dairy creams which contain 1700 and 1600 calories a pint respectively.

Milk is recognised as being a major cause of food allergies (see Chapter 4), and for this reason you may do well to try and eliminate it completely. If you do not like the natural, milk-free flavour of coffee or tea, perhaps it is time to consider a substitute (see Chapter 16).

Low-fat spread for butter

The first thing that must be said is that all vegetable margarines contain the same amount of calories as butter: 210 per 1 oz/25 g. Low-fat spreads that contain around 110 calories per 1 oz/25 g are available. In order to find which of all of the low-fat spreads that are available actually contain the least calories requires a considerable portion of the time you spend food shopping, just reading the labels. Whatever spread you finally decide on, try using half the amount that you would normally use and eliminate it completely from sandwiches. Mustard adds zip to most sandwiches, and because it is so strong you need only the tiniest amount. One level teaspoon is about 10 calories. Because they contain water, low-fat spreads and hydrogenated margarines are not suitable for cooking.

Low-fat cheese for hard and cottage cheeses
Cheese is a very concentrated form of dairy product, and that makes it high in fat. Even what seems the smallest amount can add up calories quickly. Just 1 oz/25 g of Cheddar is 117 calories. The same amount of cream cheese is 125 calories. 1 oz/25 g of plain cottage cheese, on the other hand, is only 27 calories. Low-fat cheeses are available but as the calorie count differs from product to product careful label reading is required. Low-fat Cheddar cheeses average about 75 calories per ounce. For slimming purposes it is best to avoid all except cottage cheese.

Lean meat for fatty meat
Excess calories aside, the evidence of the need to cut down on the consumption of meat – particularly fatty and red meats – has mounted to such an extent that it has become pretty difficult for anyone to ignore (see Chapter 7). Reducing meat meals to no more than once or twice a week can have a positive effect on your diet, health and wallet. That is providing, of course, that good substitutions are made. For further information on sensible substitutions, see Chapter 16. The growing trend towards vegetarianism has brought into most bookshops a whole array of wonderful vegetarian cookbooks, packed with excellent recipes, many of which require minimal time to prepare. When red meat is part of the meal it should be as lean as possible and preferably organic beef or lamb. Skin should be removed from chicken before cooking to eliminate the major part of the fat. When you do serve meat it should be minus the gravy. If you are using a really lean cut there should not be enough

leftover fat for gravy anyway.

Fish is an excellent replacement for meat and relatively low in calories, especially if it is grilled. There are a number of toppings that can be used with fish that are also low in calories as well as being tasty. Lemon can be mixed with one or more herbs (dill, basil, oregano, parsley). Garlic and onions also go well and can be chopped up and grilled on top of the fish.

Fruit for chocolates, boiled sweets, other confectionery
Between-meal snacks are very often made up of items containing a high sugar content. Because these products are advertised as being energy boosting, just the right thing for a quick pick-me-up, it seems the logical choice, and besides, they taste good. By choosing a chocolate bar, packet of biscuits, can of cola or anything with a high sugar content, you are feeding yourself high calories and energy without any nutrients – empty calories. These between-meal snacks easily become habit forming and so before you know it you are having a piece of pastry mid-morning, a chocolate bar or other confectionery and cola mid-afternoon and a late evening snack – every day. Aside from the unnecessary added calories, you are forcing your body to leach vitamins and minerals from its own store in order to digest the refined carbohydrates.

It is true that sugar from refined carbohydrates will raise the blood sugar level, but this is only a temporary phenomenon and when it falls it does so rapidly (see Hypoglycaemia, Chapter 4). It makes more sense to eat foods that contain natural sugars, such as fruit. Natural carbohydrates 'burn slower' during the digestive process and so are less likely to create the energy highs and lows that are associated with the consumption of refined sugar. In addition, fruit contains other important nutrients.

A medium-sized apple weighs about 5 oz/125 g and is approximately 50 calories. In comparison, one bourbon cream biscuit is 60 calories (and how many people can eat just one?) and a 1 oz/25 g packet of potato crisps averages at about 130 calories; the apple is clearly the more sensible choice. It is surprising how quickly one habit can be exchanged for another. By substituting fresh fruit for those between-meal snacks you can do something beneficial for your body and cut down on calories at the same time. It takes time, however: the less refined sugar that you eat the less you want to eat it. In the end it is worth the initial sacrifice as far as weight *and* health are concerned.

Baked potato or oven chips for fried chips
One of the most popular foods is probably chips or French fries. 1 oz/25 g yields approximately 72 calories as compared to 24 calories for the same weight of potato baked. The extra 48 calories per ounce is the fat that is absorbed as a result of frying; this means that 66% of the calories in chips comes from the fat they are fried in, and this is often saturated fat and/or fat that has been reused a number of times.

Baked potatoes on their own are very low in calories and make an excellent food for slimmers, as long as they are not loaded with toppings. It is the butter (210 calories per 1 oz/ 25 g), soured cream (58 per 1 oz/25 g), and cheese (Cheddar, for example, is 117 per 1 oz/25 g) that hike up the calorie count. Low-fat plain yoghurt makes a good alternative topping at only 15 calories per 1 oz/25 g and various herbs and spices can be included for added flavour. A few examples include dill, oregano and basil. For a non-fat alternative to chips, see Chapter 8.

Baked, grilled or stir fried for fried foods
Because of the added fat it produces, frying should be avoided for all foods, not just potatoes. This is not only true when weight loss is a consideration but for general health purposes as well. (One Welsh centenarian, asked what he

put his longevity down to, said, 'I'm no friend of the frying pan.') There are a number of alternative ways to prepare food that do not involve frying (see Chapter 8). And, as so often is the case, foods and food preparations that are recommended for weight loss are also good for your health.

Now have a look, if you have not already done so, at the healthy eating suggestions offered in Chapter 8.

A LOOK AT LIFESTYLE

While you are changing some of your food habits why not make a few other changes as well? In addition to burning off calories, exercise is good for increasing lung efficiency; it also loosens up your body, a positive step towards reducing stress of the physical kind. If you are not used to exercising you can always start by walking more. Swimming is excellent because it works so many muscles in the body. (See Chapter 5 for other exercise suggestions). The interesting thing about exercising is that once you really get into it you will not want to stop because of the way it will make you feel so much better.

Here are some helpful hints that should help you stick to your food plan and obtain your desired results:

Plan your daily menu in advance. You should be sure that you have all the necessary ingredients on hand. In this way you will know exactly how much to eat and you will not be forced to make costly calorie substitutes at the last minute. Consider what nutritional benefits are provided by each of your food choices. Remember, the less complex the food (raw fruits and vegetables, for example) the fewer calories they contain and the easier it is to keep an accurate calorie count. Try to concentrate on what you can eat rather than what you cannot eat.

Incorporate into your diet foods that you enjoy eating. If you only enjoy eating high calorie foods then choose the least offensive and occasionally allow yourself a small portion. You will find that there are healthy lower calorie alternatives for most high calorie foods as mentioned above and in Chapters 8 and 16, so do try substituting. You may even find that you like the alternatives better!

Before starting your meal sit back and take a few deep breaths. This will help you rid yourself of any excess tension. You may prefer a brief meditation in order to focus on the nutritional value of the food that you are about to eat. This is not far from the idea of grace before a meal. Some people repeat the procedure after their meal as well.

Allow sufficient time for each meal. It is preferable to have meals without any visual disturbances such as sitting in front of a TV set. Chewing each mouthful carefully aids digestion. Eating slowly helps to control the amount of food that you consume. Put your utensil down between each mouthful. It can take up to 20 minutes from the time you start eating for your stomach to let you know that it is full. Obviously, the faster you eat, the more probable it is that you consume more food than is required to satisfy hunger.

When you find yourself in the kitchen searching for a snack, stop and ask yourself if you are really hungry. If the desire for food has come because you are bored, depressed or any one of a thousand other reasons, try first sitting down and taking 10 really deep breaths, slowly. Rethink the situation and if you still must have something to put into your mouth, grab a carrot stick. You should have these readily available in the fridge alongside celery sticks for just such occasions. You will find some additional ideas that you may want to use in Chapter 6.

▶ GO TO ▶   ● *Quick loss technique, page 73.*
              ♦ *Diet groups and 'wonder' diets, page 151.*

11 *Keeping to a diet*

Never go shopping, especially to the supermarket, to purchase food on an empty stomach. There are sure to be more items in your trolley or basket by the time you get to the check-out counter than you intended! These items usually tend not to be of the healthy variety either. Also, be sure to avoid buying any high-calorie foods that you find irresistible, even if your family enjoys them, especially if they are not dieting with you. Shop with your head, not your tummy.

When you read food labels, be sure you understand what all the ingredients are. Remember that just because they appear further down the list this does not mean that they are not present in amounts that are significant enough to matter — it could be just the opposite. For example, there are a number of different forms in which sugar can be found (see below). If a product includes sugar from a number of different sources and the manufacturer chooses to list each separately, it could give the illusion of less sugar than is actually in the product. Remember that if a food is described as high energy it probably means that it is high in calories because calories are the units by which energy is measured.

Whether you are in the process of losing weight or not, it is important to read the nutritional information on pre-packaged foods very carefully. Some products will show the nutritional contents of the entire package while others will indicate a particular amount (4 oz/100 g, or 1 portion, which equals, say, half the pack). If a package weighs 12 oz/350 g but the nutritional information is given for 4 oz/100 g, you may be taking in more than you bargained for, calories included.

SIMPLE CALORIE-CUTTING

It is not so much the potato that adds the calories as the butter or cream you put on it! The same applies to pasta. In itself, pasta, especially wholegrain, provides protein, carbohydrates, vitamins B_1 and B_6, niacin, iron, zinc and fibre, with little fat. It is the ingredients of the sauce you cover it with that makes the difference to your calorie intake.

Whenever you feel the need for a snack, stick to one on the list of suggested snacks in Chapter 8. Many producers of high-calorie delights (chocolate, salted peanuts, etc.) package mini-versions of their products. Although these may contain fewer calories because of their size, it does not change the fact that most of these products have minimal (if any) nutritional value. And besides, can you really be satisfied with just one? Better to avoid them completely.

Most people do not realise just how many foods contain added sugar, nor how much. (An average tablespoon of tomato ketchup contains about one teaspoon of sugar, for example!) Most ingredient lists on packaging will contain sugar in some form, so it is necessary to be familiar with all of the variations. These include dextrose, glucose, maltose, fructose, sucrose, maple syrup, honey and corn syrup (see Chapter 14). On top of all this, people add yet more sugar to tea, coffee, cereals, desserts ...

EATING OUT

Eating out can be hazardous to your health in more ways than one, particularly if the restaurant choice is one of the fast food variety. Some fast food chains have started to add items that have more nutritional value to the menu. The fact still remains that unless you know exactly what is in the food you could be taking in a lot of unnecessary calories and unfavourable additives as well. According to Dr Tim Lobstein of the London Food Commission, some fast food chains include sugar in chips, monosodium glutamate in chicken nuggets and cold ham, and animal fats (saturated) in pizza, buns and chips. Excessive use of salt is another concern. If you are purchasing a meal from a fast food chain, or any restaurant for that matter, you have a right to know what ingredients are being used. It may be their prerogative not to want to divulge such information, but ultimately it is your prerogative whether or not you eat there.

Eating out need not be a problem even when you are trying to lose weight, providing you follow a few simple ground rules:

Try to bring your own lunch (or supper) to work. By preparing it ahead of time you eliminate the risk of not having enough time just before leaving for work. Be sure to include fresh fruit which can be eaten as a snack at coffee break time.

Favour fish. When eating out cannot be avoided, grilled fish is a good choice. Even if grilled fish is not a choice on the menu, as long as fish is, any good restaurant should be able to specially prepare it for you. Make sure you emphasise that you do not want it made with butter, or any sauce for that matter, just a slice of fresh lemon. Choose a baked potato, again without any added butter or other calorie-ridden toppings. With the addition of a side salad, you have a nutritious, low-calorie meal. For non-meat eaters, a baked potato and a large salad is a good choice. Salad dressing can be a problem, particularly the cream variety, and so it might not be a bad idea to bring your own! A quick dressing can be prepared by combining freshly squeezed lemon or apple cider vinegar with a number of herbs (see below). You need just a small amount so a bottle of the mixture can easily be tucked into a handbag or even a pocket.

FOOD PREPARATION TIPS

An easy way to cook grains like couscous, millet and barley is to cover the food with twice as much water as grain, bring to a boil, place the lid on, remove from the heat and let stand for at least 25 minutes. Vegetables like artichoke can also be cooked in this manner.

When substituting honey for sugar in a recipe, in addition to using between only ⅓ and ½ of the specified amount, be sure to reduce the total amount of liquid by ¼ of the amount of honey used.

SPICING UP A DIET

Much can be done to relatively unexciting foods to turn them into appetising delights and keep them low in calories at the same time. The secret is knowing what herbs and spices to use. Spices are basically the dried aromatic parts of plants and each has its own characteristic flavour. Herbs are seed plants in that they do not develop permanent woody tissue and do not last beyond a single growing season. Many plants seem to overlap the two definitions and so for the purpose of this book they will be considered the same.

In addition, it should be mentioned that certain spices such as fennel and mint are known to aid digestion and traditionally have been used by many cultures for that purpose in addition to the wonderful flavours they provide. For easy reference Table 6 lists various foods and the spices which go well with them.

Table 6: Foods and suitable accompanying herbs and spices

Herbs and spices can be used in sauces, soups, salads, casseroles and with all types of food including vegetables, meats, grains, dairy produce, fish and poultry. They can be used with just about anything, savoury or sweet dishes. Below are 36 spices and herbs with some suggestions for foods to use them with.

Flavouring herb or spice:	*Foods to use with:*
Basil	Salads, vegetables (tomatoes, peppers, aubergines), tomato sauce, eggs
Bay leaves	Marinades, pickles, soups, sauces
Capers	Salads, pizza, meat sauces, fish sauces
Caraway seeds	Carrots, soups, bread, sweet cakes and biscuits
Cardamom	Rice, other grains, cakes, pastries, poultry
Cayenne pepper	Seafood, cheese, vegetables, soups, casseroles, sauces, dips
Celery seed	Soups, dips, sauces, salads, tomato
Chilli powder	Tomato sauce, curry, meat, fish, seafood
Chives	Sour cream, cottage cheese, cucumber, potato, eggs, soups
Cinnamon	Desserts of all kinds, rice pudding, apples, on toast, savoury dishes, curry, spiced wine
Cloves	Sweet yellow vegetables, apple sauce, baked beans, fruit compotes, curry, meat casseroles, spiced wine
Coriander	Meat, fish, vegetables, curry, tomato sauce, poultry
Cumin	Rice, other grains, fish, meat, curry, yoghurt, vegetables, poultry

Table 6: Foods and suitable accompanying herbs and spices (continued)

Curry powder	Meat, fish, curry, vegetables, relishes
Dill	Potatoes (hot or cold), pickling, soup, sauces, cakes, fish, poultry, stuffing, meat, vegetables, sour cream, yoghurt
Fennel	Fish, soup, sauces, cakes, bread, curry
Fenugreek	Chutney, pickles, vegetables, lentils, salads, yoghurt
Garlic	Almost everything savoury, meats, fish, vegetables, on bread, soups, sauces, casseroles, salads
Ginger	Baked beans, fish, meat, vegetables, curry, cakes, biscuits, sauces, jams, fruit compote, ice cream
Mint	Tea, mint sauce, jam, desserts, peas, potatoes, cucumbers, fruit compote
Mustard	Salads, sauces, baked beans, curry, meat, fish, vegetables, relish
Nutmeg	Green vegetables, apple sauce, eggs, desserts, cheese, spiced wine
Oregano	Tomato sauces, soups, casseroles, pasta
Paprika	Poultry, soups, sauces, vegetables, meats, shellfish, eggs, cheese
Parsley	Fish, meat, vegetables, sauces, salads, eggs
Pepper	Savoury dishes, meats, poultry, fish, vegetables, soups, casseroles
Rosemary	Poultry, lamb, green beans, spinach
Saffron	Rice, other grains, rice pudding, cake and buns, seafood, fish
Sage	Meat, fish, stuffing

Table 6: Foods and suitable accompanying herbs and spices (continued)

Sesame seed	Bread, cakes, tahini, hummus, stir-fried dishes, casseroles
Shallot	Soups, sauces, salads, casseroles, meat, fish, vegetables, quiches
Tarragon	Salads, poultry, fish, eggs, salads, sauces
Thyme	Soups, marinades, stuffing, vegetables, fish, cheese, meat, poultry
Turmeric	Meat, fish, vegetables, curry, eggs, sauces, rice, other grains
Vanilla	All desserts, fruits
Watercress	Salads, soups, casseroles

Note: Tofu goes well with all of the above spices and herbs.

Further information can be found in an excellent book which provides an abundance of information, *Spices and Natural Flavourings,* by Jennifer Mulherin.

▶ GO TO ▶   ♦ *Nutrients, vitamins and minerals, page 157.*

12 Diets to combat disease

Most of the diet suggestions listed in this book are compiled from a number of sources. References are given in the Bibliography. Where specific diets are outlined, as in the case of the Bristol Diet, contact information is provided. (Please remember to include a stamp for return postage when requesting information from any of the organisations listed in this book. Many of these groups are non-profitmaking and in any case it will be appreciated.)

In all cases, where diet suggestions are made, these are intended as guidelines only. Further information should always be sought from a qualified health practitioner or appropriate centre. Where important nutrients are indicated it is suggested that emphasis be placed on including foods that contain these nutrients in your diet. Supplements should be taken under the guidance of a qualified practitioner.

In addition to a proper balanced diet, it is also important to consider exercise and stress control techniques. Research shows that in most of the diseases discussed in this book, both stress and inadequate exercise play a part.

Chapters 8 and 10 provide the basis for a balanced healthy diet and this is suggested as the foundation for all the diseases discussed below. Many of the chapters in Part Three (Further Information) also contribute valuable information to assist you in making good product choices. The following dietary advice is intended to provide guidance and includes foods that are potentially beneficial or detrimental to each disease. In all cases, try to obtain the necessary nutrients from food sources and if supplements are used, do not exceed the recommended dose.

Acne

Fibre intake should be increased to aid the elimination process.

Foods to avoid/restrict:
- all refined carbohydrates (white flour, sugar, etc.);
- fried foods;
- milk and milk products (high hormone content);
- foods containing hydrogenated vegetable oils (margarine).

Acquired immunodeficiency syndrome (AIDS)

It appears that a dysfunctioning immune system may be at the root of this disease. A decrease in potential allergy causing foods could alleviate some of the stress placed upon the immune system.

Foods to avoid/restrict:
- refined carbohydrates (white bread, white flour, etc);
- meat and dairy products (saturated fats).

Recommended foods:
- complex carbohydrates/high fibre/low fat;
- moderate amounts of protein;
- garlic (good for immune system).

Important nutrients:
- vitamin A – supports immune system;
- vitamin C – supports immune system and inhibits viruses;
- zinc – supports the immune system.

Alzheimer's disease

Replacement of aluminium utensils and food containers by other materials such as glass or stainless steel (although more expensive) will avoid leaching of aluminium into foods. The high level of aluminium found in many deodorants and drugs such as antacids should also be considered.

Foods to restrict/avoid;
• tap water for drinking may include high levels of various substances, including aluminium, and should be checked (see Chapter 18);
• processed foods packaged in aluminium.

Recommended foods:
• complex carbohydrates/high fibre/low fat;
• moderate amounts of protein;
• mineral water.

Important nutrients:
• vitamin B12 – deficiencies associated with dementia;
• vitamins C and E – natural antioxidant which prevents damage from free radicals (see Glossary of terms);
• zinc – helps normalise immune defects.

Arthritis
A detoxification programme (see Chapter 8) should be considered as a possible first step in conjunction with an elimination diet (Chapter 4) as food allergy may be linked with arthritis.

Foods to restrict/avoid:
• all refined carbohydrates;
• meat and dairy products;
• foods from nightshade (*Solanceae*) family (aubergine, peppers, white potatoes, tomatoes) – may promote inflammation of the joints;
• salt;
• sugar;
• coffee, tea, cola drinks;
• chocolate.

Recommended foods:
• complex carbohydrates/high fibre/low fat;
• cold water fish (mackerel, herring, salmon, sardines);
• chicken without skin and preferably free range;

- sprouts (alfalfa, mung, etc.);
- fresh vegetable juice;
- cherries, blackberries, etc.

Important nutrients:
- vitamin B-complex – important in the functioning of the nervous system. Good for muscle tone and joint mobility;
- vitamin C – essential for healthy bones, tendons and cartilage;
- vitamin E – acts as an antioxidant;
- calcium – promotes tone and elasticity of soft joint tissues;
- magnesium – enhances ability to contract muscles;
- manganese – aids in proper functioning of collagen;
- selenium – reduces production of inflammatory leukotrienes (see Asthma);
- zinc – aids calcium metabolism and helps heal irritated tissues.

Asthma

A trial elimination of animal products may be appropriate as the stimulation of bronchial constriction can be caused by leukotrienes, substances which are produced by the body and are derived from a fatty acid found only in animal products (see vegan diet, Chapter 15).

Foods to restrict/avoid:
- coffee and tea;
- chocolate;
- refined carbohydrates – particularly sugar and white flour;
- processed foods – these often contain refined carbohydrates;
- additives, colouring and saturated fats (read labels carefully);
- animal proteins – meat and dairy products;
- excessive salt intake;

• alcohol.

Recommended foods:
• complex carbohydrates/high fibre/low fat;
• moderate protein;
• garlic and onions - inhibits manufacture of leuko-trienes;
• cayenne pepper - helps restrict swelling of sinus passages;
• spring water - at least 2 pints/1200 ml daily.

Important nutrients:
• vitamins B6, B12, C, E;
• carotene (vitamin A), selenium, magnesium.

Atherosclerosis (heart/stroke)
There is little doubt that low-density lipoprotein (LDL) cholesterol build-up is one of the leading factors in the cause of atherosclerosis. It is also true that cholesterol is vital for life function. The body produces its own choles-terol and so a reduction in the amount we obtain from our food, in particular saturated fats, would seem appropriate. A modified vegetarian diet could be considered (see Chap-ter 15).

Foods to restrict/avoid:
• saturated fats - meats, eggs and dairy products. When eating meat it is important to eliminate as much fat as possible;
• calamari - along with caviar, the only fish foods that should be restricted because of high cholesterol and fat content;
• added salt - excessive salt can cause high blood pressure - it is important to read labels as salt is added to many processed foods;
• coffee;
• alcohol;
• fried foods.

Recommended foods:
- fish – particularly mackerel, salmon, sardines and herring;
- high-fibre foods – particularly oat bran which is high in water-soluble fibre, which helps lower cholesterol levels. Rice bran and barley are other good choices;
- fresh vegetables and fruits – broccoli and cauliflower can help lower cholesterol, and pectin (from apples and grapefruit) is also good;
- whole grain products;
- beans and pulses – aids in lowering of cholesterol levels;
- linseed oil – one of the best sources of linolenic acid;
- brewer's yeast – rich in chromium which helps decrease LDL cholesterol while increasing HDL levels;
- garlic and onions – cholesterol lowering effects;
- ginger – lowers cholesterol levels and helps prevent blood clots;
- alfalfa – decreases cholesterol and arterial plaque.

Important nutrients:
- vitamin B3 (niacin) – helps lower cholesterol levels;
- folic acid – a B vitamin that is good for blood flow;
- vitamin C – helps cholesterol metabolism;
- vitamin E (and selenium) – helps control free radicals;
- evening primrose oil – helps in lowering cholesterol levels;
- calcium – helps decrease serum cholesterol;
- copper – important in the production of connective tissue;
- lecithin (polyunsaturated forms only) – aids in removal of cholesterol from tissue deposits;
- magnesium – helps protect against atherosclerosis.

Cancer – the Bristol diet
The Bristol Cancer Help Centre in Bristol received much publicity in 1991 because of a study that was conducted

there which concluded that women with breast cancer 'are likely to fare worse' as a result of going to the Centre. The report (in the *Lancet*) was quickly picked up by the media and became headline material, a topic for TV news reports and two BBC special programmes. What was not as heavily covered was the change of mind that occurred when the report was later questioned. It appears that the details of patients who had only visited the clinic on one occasion were included in the statistics. Whether they actually followed any of the advice they may have received was an unknown factor. People who went to the Centre tended to have more advanced conditions than those using orthodox treatment. In order for a study to have any meaning it must compare like with like, and this study clearly did not. A sort of retraction was later published in the *Lancet* by the research team, but to my knowledge this was not picked up by the popular press.

The diet that the Bristol Cancer Help Centre prescribes is designed to cleanse the system of toxic substances while building up the body's natural self-healing ability. An outline of the Bristol Diet approach is as follows:

• no meat – the necessary protein is obtained from vegetables, fruit and whole-grain cereals;
• low protein – this is in order not to overwork that part of the pancreas that produces enzymes which work to allow the digestion of protein. The idea is to allow the enzymes produced by the pancreas to concern themselves with destroying cancerous tumours (which are coated with protein) rather than having to concentrate too much of their efforts on protein intake as a result of a high protein diet. The Bristol Diet is thus designed to allow for enough protein to stimulate the pancreas into enzyme production without causing all of the enzymes produced to have to deal with protein intake. This allows some of the enzymes the opportunity to work on breaking down the protein-coated

cancer cells;

• approximately 70% of food should be eaten raw. This eliminates the destruction of important vitamins and enzymes during the cooking process. Grated raw vegetables (vegetables can be juiced for patients who have a problem with swallowing) form the most important part of each meal;

• sprouted beans, seeds and grains are a good source of vitamins and enzymes;

• no processed foods of any kind;

• no tea or coffee;

• additional vitamins and minerals, in the form of supplements, are given where necessary.

Further information on the Bristol Cancer Help Centre may be obtained from: 7 Downfield Road, Clifton, Bristol BS8 2TG, telephone (0272) 743216.

Candida diet

This diet is aimed primarily at eliminating foods which promote the growth of *Candida albicans* while providing foods which contain nutrients beneficial for the immune system.

Foods to avoid:

• all forms of sugar – sugar encourages yeast overgrowth (includes honey, molasses, maple syrup, sugar substitutes, alcoholic drinks);

• gluten (wheat, rye, oats, barley) – the presence of candida inhibits the digestion of gluten;

• foods containing yeasts and moulds (bread, vinegar, pickled foods, sauces such as ketchup and Worcestershire, mushrooms, cheese, spices, alcohol, fruit, malted products, monosodium glutamate, peanuts, pistachios, other nuts unless they are very fresh, meat, coffee, tea, including herbal teas);

• fruit should be avoided initially because of its high natural sugar content, and eaten in moderation when reintroduced to the diet. An exception is melon, which should not be eaten because its porous skin makes it a candidate for mould;

• fruit juices – these can contain mould if the fruit has been left in holding bins for any length of time prior to being processed;

• milk and milk products (milk has a high content of lactose – milk sugar – in addition to trace levels of antibiotics);

• soft drinks — these contain caffeine, food colouring, phosphates;

• artificial sweeteners;

• refined carbohydrates – an ingredient of nearly all processed foods.

Recommended foods:

• fresh vegetables (organically grown where possible);

• lamb, wild game, poultry (free range where possible);

• small quantities of fruit (none during the first few weeks);

• fresh nuts (from the shell) and seeds;

• beans and non-gluten grains (millet, rice, corn);

• yoghurt (only live culture contains *Lactobacillus acidophilus* which retards candida growth);

• eggs (free range where possible);

• seafood;

• a diet rich in essential fatty acids. These are necessary to help regulate many body processes. Sources for EFAs include cold-pressed linseed oil, spinach, kale, parsley, green peppers, fish oils from salmon, sardines and mackerel;

• garlic (for its antifungal activity);

• spices – cinnamon, ginger, lemon balm, rosemary, thyme.

Important nutrients:
• vitamin B-complex, vitamin C and zinc are all important for the immune system.

Further information on candida may also be obtained from the ME Action Campaign (see Useful addresses).

Cystitis
With this condition it is important to drink large amounts of fluids, including unsweetened cranberry juice, to keep the urinary tract flushed.

Foods to restrict/avoid:
• simple sugars – for their detrimental effect on the immune system;
• refined carbohydrates;
• full-strength fruit juices.

Recommended foods:
• unsweetened cranberry juice – this reduces the ability of bacteria to adhere to the bladder lining and urethra;
• garlic – helpful in fighting diseases;
• onion.

Important nutrients:
• vitamins A and C;
• zinc.

Diabetes
The dietary recommendations outlined here are those of the British Diabetic Association; comments, where appropriate, have been included in brackets.

Recommended foods:
• maintain as even a calorie intake as possible from day to day;
• eat regular meals;
• half the calories should come from starchy high fibre

carbohydrate foods (wholemeal bread, jacket potatoes, brown rice, wholegrain pasta and cereals, beans and lentils. Foods rich in vitamin E are important as this vitamin appears to help normalise insulin release from the pancreas and is helpful in circulatory problems which are common to diabetics);

• beans, lentils, oats and citrus fruits should be eaten often as they create a slow and steady rise in blood glucose (oat bran helps maintain a normal glucose level in addition to lowering cholesterol);

• eat less sugar – this includes sweetened soft drinks, cakes, sweets, chocolates, keeping them only for special occasions (it might be better, however, to eliminate them completely);

• cut down on fat intake – eat less fatty red meat and meat products – replace with fish and poultry (eliminate skin from poultry before cooking and use free range when possible);

• use low fat spread in place of butter or margarine;

• use skimmed or semi-skimmed milk rather than whole milk (again it might be better to try a soya milk substitute or eliminate completely);

• cut down on salt – found in pre-cooked meats, smoked fish and cheese which have a high salt content (enough salt is found naturally in foods and so the elimination of the salt shaker from the table might be a good idea);

• use low fat yoghurt; save cream for special occasions (as long as special occasions do not happen too often – also, ensure that the yoghurt used is live culture in order to obtain any benefit from it);

• choose low-calorie soft drinks (or better still, stick to mineral water);

• tinned fruit in natural juice rather than syrup (best of all, go for fresh fruit only);

• for recipes containing sugar, use half the amount (or substitute honey or raw molasses in small amounts);

• substitute an intense sweetener – such as aspartame – instead of sugar (better still, eliminate completely);
• cut down on salty crisps and other salty snacks (here you could substitute the word 'out' for 'down');
• limit alcohol consumption;
• avoid special diabetic foods – these are usually low in fibre.

In an article in the April/May 1989 issue of *Balance* (the journal produced by the British Diabetic Association) entitled 'Diabetic Foods Do We Need Them?', it was stated that 'Diabetic foods are lower in sugar than ordinary foods ... are generally no lower in fat or calories than ordinary equivalents ... have little health benefit.' Basically, these special foods offer little advantage over their ordinary counterparts and are generally higher in price. It would make more sense to eat more raw foods and eliminate processed foods altogether.

The British Diabetic Association has been in existence for over 50 years and concerns itself with fund raising for research. They produce a number of publications. *Balance* is produced bi-monthly. An information pack produced by the British Diabetic Association is also available (see Useful addresses).

Eczema
Since food allergy is considered to be a leading cause of eczema, it is, of course, important to determine which food(s) are involved. Although this can differ from individual to individual, there are certain foods which seem to be the main triggers. The most logical approach would be an elimination diet as discussed in Chapter 4.

Common food allergens:
• cow's milk – the first food protein normally given to infants and the food source which most commonly triggers eczema;

• eggs – high protein content provides stimulus;
• all animal products – this includes meats, poultry, and all dairy products (butter, cheese, etc.). It is important to remember that many carbohydrates (bread, cakes, etc.) contain dairy products;
• wheat – usually due to gluten;
• foods containing artificial colourings and preservatives – particularly azo colourings and benzoate preservatives (see Chapter 17).

Suggested replacement foods for those eliminated:
• soya 'milk' (a nutritionally complete soya milk formula specifically designed for infants is available);
• casein hydrolysate formula (made from cow's milk but altered to remove allergenic proteins);
• egg substitutes may be used but it is important to read labels as some may contain ovalbumin, an egg protein;
• rye, corn, barley or potato flour may be used instead of wheat;
• foods that do not contain any artificial colouring or preservatives;
• fish oils (particularly mackerel, herring and salmon which are all high in EPA).

Important vitamins and minerals:
• vitamin A (for the development and maintenance of skin);
• zinc (necessary for the enzyme that produces hydro-chloric acid in the stomach and necessary in converting fatty acids to anti-inflammatory prostaglandins).

Further information may be obtained from the National Eczema Society (see Useful addresses).

Food allergies
A simple test for a potential food allergy using a variation of the elimination diet technique would be to keep a record

of everything you eat. At the same time keep a parallel record and indicate at what points the particular chronic symptom you are testing for occurred. By cross referencing the two lists it may be possible to see if there is a correlation between a certain food(s) and a flare up of the symptoms. The next step would be to eliminate the food from the diet for a period of six days. It is most important to remember that all foods that contain the particular potential allergen must also be eliminated. In the case of wheat that would mean such items as cake, biscuits and bread. Careful label reading of products is essential. If a particular product does not have a list of ingredients, write to the manufacturer requesting one. Foods belonging to the same botanic group should also be considered. Wheat, for example, belongs to the same botanic group as rye, barley, rice, oats, malt, corn and cane sugar. If symptoms are alleviated, it is best to stay away from the allergen. Often, however, food allergies are difficult to ascertain precisely, especially when a sensitivity to more than one food exists. In addition, because each person is biochemically individual, diet needs and restrictions can also be different in each case even though the illness or food allergy is the same.

A more complex elimination diet is best done under the guidance of a qualified nutritionist.

Common food allergens:
• cow's milk – and related products such as cheese and eggs;
• wheat – the gluten is the most common part causing allergy;
• foods containing histamine – preserves, sauerkraut, sausage, spinach, tomato, tuna, wine;
• foods that release histamine – chocolate, strawberry, tomato, shellfish, alcohol;
• citrus fruits.

Food recommendations:
• organic, chemical/hormone free foods.

A four-day rotation diet (developed by Dr Herbert Rinkel in 1934) should be considered, particularly for those more prone to food allergy, to avoid creating any new allergies which can occur as a result of eating a food too often. Of course any known food allergens should automatically be eliminated, at least initially. It may, however, be possible to reintroduce them back into the diet after a period of time. Space is limited here but there are a number of excellent books available that deal with this subject – two are *An Alternative Approach To Allergies* by T G Randolph and R W Moss, and *Coping With Your Allergies* by N and F G Golos (see Bibliography).

Important nutrients:
• vitamin A, B-complex – helpful to the immune system;
• selenium – helpful to the immune system;
• zinc – helpful to the immune system;
• vitamin C – antihistaminic properties;
• evening primrose oil and fish oils – increase anti-inflammatory prostaglandin production.

For further information contact Action Against Allergy, (see Useful addresses).

Gallstones
A diet low in fibre and high in refined carbohydrates and fats will cause a decrease in the amount of bile acids produced by the liver, which can lead to the formation of gall stones. Excess cholesterol will cause the same problem.

If food allergy is suspected, an elimination diet may be appropriate (see Chapter 4).

Foods to restrict/avoid:
• refined carbohydrates;

- sugar;
- saturated fats;
- animal protein (meat, cheese, milk, etc. – sources of cholesterol);
- all fried foods.

Dietary recommendations:
- a vegetarian diet may be beneficial (see Chapter 15);
- complex carbohydrates/high fibre/low fat;
- soya products;
- fresh vegetables (high fibre – aids in reversal as well as prevention);
- fresh fruit (fibre-rich to aid in reversal and prevention);
- oat bran;
- linseed;
- six to eight glasses of spring water daily.

Important nutrients:
- vitamins C and E (deficiency may contribute to the cause of gallstones).

Gout

It is important to reduce the amount of purine-containing foods (purines form the compound found in uric acid) in order to decrease the concentration of uric acid which forms the crystals that are then deposited in the joints. A diet low in fat and protein is recommended. It is also important to ensure liberal amounts of fluid intake, which increases the excretion of uric acid.

Obesity is common among gout sufferers. A diet designed to incorporate slimming techniques and guidelines may be required (see Chapters 5 and 10).

Foods to restrict/avoid:
- purine-containing foods (meat – particularly organ meats, yeast, poultry, shellfish, herring, sardines, mackerel, anchovies, pulses);

- fats – particularly saturated fats as they increase uric acid retention;
- refined carbohydrates – increase uric acid production;
- sugar – provides unnecessary calories;
- alcohol – inhibits uric acid secretion.

Recommended foods:
- complex carbohydrates/high fibre/low fat;
- cherries – lower uric acid levels.

Important nutrients:
- vitamin E and selenium – acts as an antioxidant.

Hypertension (high blood pressure)
Maintaining a balanced diet is one of the best factors in prevention and cure of hypertension. Normal body weight is another important factor; this, of course, can be controlled with proper diet. A modified vegetarian diet could be considered (see Chapter 15).

Foods to avoid/restrict:
- caffeine – affects the adrenaline glands which can cause hypertension. Caffeine is found in coffee, tea, chocolate and cola drinks;
- saturated fats – meat, eggs and dairy produce;
- added salt – can damage blood pressure regulating mechanisms;
- refined carbohydrates;
- sugar – elevates blood pressure.

Recommended foods:
- high fibre whole foods – particularly those containing water soluble fibre such as oats and oat bran;
- wholefoods – grains, lentils, beans;
- fresh vegetables and fruits;
- garlic and onions – decrease blood pressure.

Important nutrients:
- calcium – blood pressure lowering effect;

- magnesium – blood pressure lowering effect;
- vitamin C – relation with blood pressure;
- potassium – it is important to maintain a proper sodium (salt) potassium balance to reduce the risk of high blood pressure;
- zinc – aids in reducing hypertension.

Hypoglycaemia

The common consensus is that excessive consumption of refined carbohydrates (particularly sugar and white flour) is the leading cause of hypoglycaemia.

It has been suggested that meals with smaller portions should be eaten more frequently than the standard three times a day. Rather than grabbing a chocolate bar when hit with a feeling of between-meal hunger, a piece of fruit or a handful of nuts (the unsalted, non-dry roasted kind) would be more appropriate.

Foods to restrict/avoid:
- refined carbohydrates (especially sugar and white flour) – excessive amounts of sugar overstimulates the pancreas;
- saturated fats – meat and dairy products;
- processed foods – usually contain refined carbohydrates and saturated fats.

Recommended foods:
- fruits and vegetables – preferably organic with a high percentage eaten raw;
- garlic – rejuvenating effect on body;
- complex carbohydrates/high fibre/low fat.

Irritable bowel syndrome (IBS)

An increase in dietary fibre is of primary importance. However, because wheat is commonly used as a source of fibre, and as it has been suggested that food allergy may play a part in IBS, it may be a good idea to consider an elimination diet (see Chapter 4) which excludes wheat products since wheat is one of the most common causes of food allergy.

Foods to restrict/avoid:
• individual food sensitivities;
• refined carbohydrates.

Recommended foods:
• high fibre – particularly vegetables, fruits, oat bran, pulses;
• peppermint tea – peppermint is effective in relieving flatulence;
• ginger – effective in relieving flatulence.

Kidney stones
Excess calcium in the diet is one of the reasons for the formation of kidney stones. A diet high in protein (mainly derived from animal products) is therefore not advisable. A vegetarian diet (see Chapter 15) reduces the risk of kidney stones.

Foods to restrict/avoid:
• refined carbohydrates – very often contain milk and eggs;
• milk – very often fortified with vitamin D, which not only results in lower magnesium levels but also increases the absorption of calcium, increasing the urinary calcium concentration;
• reduction of foods high in oxalate such as: black tea, cocoa, spinach, beet leaves, rhubarb, parsley, cranberry and nuts;
• other animal protein (meat and dairy products) – these contain high levels of protein.

Recommended foods:
• foods with high magnesium/calcium ratio (barley, bran, corn, buckwheat, rye, soya, oats, brown rice, avocado, banana, broad beans, potato);

• fresh fruits and vegetables;
• high fibre - use wholewheat bread rather than white bread.

Important nutrients:
• magnesium - important in the prevention of kidney stones because it helps increase the solubility of calcium;
• vitamin B6 - works in conjunction with magnesium;
• vitamin K - helps inhibit calcium oxalate crystalline formation.

Migraine
Food allergy is sometimes linked with migraine. An elimination diet may be appropriate (see Chapter 4).

Foods to restrict/avoid:
• chocolate - a common precipitator of migraine;
• cheese - a common precipitator of migraine;
• alcohol (particularly red wine) - inhibits action of enzyme which is commonly lower in migraine sufferers;
• meat and animal products.

Recommended foods:
• fish (except shellfish) - decreases platelet aggregation;
• cayenne pepper - inhibits platelet aggregation;
• garlic;
• onion.

Important nutrients:
• magnesium;
• niacin;
• oil of evening primrose.

Myalgic encephalomyelitis (ME)
A detoxification programme to stimulate the liver and other organs dealing with elimination in the body should be considered (see Chapter 7).

Food allergies should also be a consideration,

particularly to wheat as a large number of ME sufferers appear to have a sensitivity to gluten.

Foods to restrict/avoid:
- saturated fats – meats and dairy products;
- refined carbohydrates – sugar, white flour, polished rice, white pasta (includes products made from these sources);
- processed foods;
- food additives, colourings, flavourings;
- fried foods;
- excessive salt intake;
- coffee, tea, soft drinks containing sugar, additives, colourings, etc.;
- chocolate;
- alcohol.

Recommended foods:
- spring water – at least eight glasses a day;
- fresh vegetables and fruits – preferably organic and raw. The best cooking method is to steam for a short period of time;
- fish – good protein source as well as providing iodine and zinc. Should be eaten at least twice a week, especially oily fish such as mackerel, sardines, tuna and herring;
- poultry – free range and organic where possible;
- free-range eggs – now widely available;
- wholegrain unprocessed foods – high in fibre and complex carbohydrates;
- pulses – good protein source;
- nuts – buy in the shell;
- herbal teas, pure unsweetened fruit juices, mineral water;
- live yoghurt – contains balancing bacteria necessary for proper function of intestines;
- garlic and onion – aids the immune system in inhibiting viruses.

Important nutrients:
• beta carotene (vitamin A) – a natural antioxidant;
• vitamin B-complex – for general health;
• vitamin C – aids in resistance to and recovery from infection;
• zinc – aids in cellular immunity;
• evening primrose oil – particularly useful for women who suffer with menstrual problems.

Further information may be obtained from ME Action Campaign (see Useful addresses).

Multiple sclerosis (MS)

As there appears to be a connection between diets rich in animal and dairy products and MS, a vegetarian or vegan diet should be considered (see Chapter 15). It is interesting that incidence of MS in Japan, where fish is consumed in much greater proportion than meat, is low.

Foods to restrict/avoid:
• meat and dairy products – high in saturated fats;
• margarine, lard, hydrogenated oils;
• sugar;
• refined carbohydrates;
• processed food.

Recommended foods:
• fresh vegetables – some raw vegetables should be eaten daily;
• fresh fruit;
• cold water fish (mackerel, salmon, herring) – should be consumed at least three times a week because they contain essential fatty acids which are important in maintaining normal nerve cell function;
• cod liver oil;
• pulses, wholegrains, vegetables – needed for protein content;
• sunflower, linseed or safflower oil for salads.

Important nutrients:
• evening primrose oil;
• selenium;
• vitamin E.

Further information may be obtained from: ARMS (Action for Research into Multiple Sclerosis) (see Useful addresses).

Osteoporosis

A number of dietary factors are implicated in the development of osteoporosis. It has been shown that excessive protein can be detrimental in this condition because it causes increased calcium loss in urine. It is also important to maintain a proper calcium/phosphorus balance (two to one seems to be satisfactory). The best calcium phosphorus ratio is found in green leafy vegetables. Research has shown that both vegetarian and vegan diets (see Chapter 15) seem to curtail the risk of osteoporosis. Proper exercise and stress reduction are also important (see *Brittle Bones and the Calcium Crisis* by Kathleen Mayes).

Foods to restrict/avoid:
• meat and dairy products – high protein sources;
• carbonated beverages – high in phosphates;
• sugar – increases the urinary excretion of calcium;
• coffee, cocoa and red wine – leaches calcium from the body.

Recommended foods:
• fruits – particularly dark-coloured berries;
• vegetables – main source of boron (see below); green leafy vegetables, which also contain vitamin K, are particularly high;
• canned salmon and sardines – good source of calcium when bones are included;
• tofu – an excellent protein source.

Important nutrients:
• vitamin B-complex – important in amino acid conversion;
• vitamin D – stimulates the absorption of calcium. The best source is from sunlight;
• vitamin K – important in bone structure;
• boron – important in hormone activation;
• calcium – important for bones;
• magnesium – particularly important if you obtain vitamin D from fortified dairy foods as they tend to decrease magnesium absorption.

Psoriasis
To eliminate the possibility of toxic build-up in either the bowels or liver, a detoxification programme may be appropriate (see Chapter 7).

Foods to avoid:
• alcohol (increases the absorption of toxins);
• meat and dairy products (high leukotriene production found in psoriasis cases);
• sugar (possible insulin insensitivity).

Recommended diets and foods:
• vegetarian or vegan diet;
• complex carbohydrates/high fibre/low fat;
• fresh fruits and vegetables (fibre essential for healthy colon);
• fish oils (high in EPA, particularly mackerel, salmon and herring);
• cider vinegar – aids digestion.

Important nutrients:
• zinc (anti-inflammatory effects);
• chromium (increases insulin receptor sensitivity);
• vitamin E (increase low co-enzyme levels);
• selenium (increase low co-enzyme levels).

Ulcers

If food allergy is suspected, an elimination diet may be appropriate (see Chapter 4). In addition, it has been found that aspirin is a gastric irritant and can cause damage to the lining of the stomach and so can actually cause the development of gastric ulcers. It would make sense to avoid the taking of aspirin if ulcers are already diagnosed.

Foods to restrict/avoid:
• milk – the most common food found to cause allergy, it has also been found to increase natural acid production, which can aid in the erosion of the stomach and duodenum linings. (*Note:* the British Digestive Foundation in their leaflet 'All About Ulcers' suggests the taking of 'soothing milky drinks or simple antacid mixtures to relieve the pain'. In the light of the increasing amount of evidence that milk is a primary cause of food allergy, and a potential irritant to ulcers, it may be wise to fully investigate this advice before adhering to it.)
• coffee (including decaffeinated).

Recommended foods:
• raw cabbage juice – long known to be effective for the treatment of peptic ulcers. Take 2 pints/1 litre daily, spread out during the course of the day;
• vegetables (especially mustard greens, turnip greens, kale, broccoli and cauliflower;
• high fibre – reduces the risk of duodenal ulcers.

Important nutrients:
• vitamins A and E;
• zinc.

Varicose veins (including haemorrhoids)

Exercise is an important part of any daily routine and this is particularly true for people suffering from varicose veins. As obesity is often associated with varicose veins, exercise is also an important part of weight loss.

Haemorrhoids are basically varicose veins of the rectum and therefore the same food considerations would apply.

Foods to restrict/avoid:
• low fibre/refined foods – causes strain/constipation.

Recommended foods:
• high fibre – to promote peristaltic movement of the bowel (vegetables, fruits, pulses, wholegrains);
• blackberries, cherries, bilberries – helps strengthen vein structure;
• onions;
• garlic;
• ginger;
• cayenne pepper – high in vitamin C.

Important nutrients:
• vitamins A, B-complex, C and E;
• zinc.

▶ GO TO ▶   ♦ *Healthy foods, page 187*

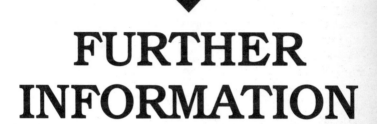

FURTHER
INFORMATION

13 *Diet groups and 'wonder' diets*

Most areas of the country have a slimming club not too far away. These are useful for those who would like the added discipline of someone else charting their progress, or who just prefer to be with others who are seeking the same goal. A number of different companies offer such services and basically the routine is the same. The group meets once a week. There is usually a joining fee in addition to the weekly fee. Each person is weighed in and a record is kept of progress. Most clubs will require that the weekly fee be paid regardless of whether you attend or not. This is done to discourage people from skipping classes for reasons such as lack of resolve or worry that a reduction of weight was not achieved or even that some was gained. Most groups do make allowances for illness or vacations, however.

A weight chart is usually employed and this will determine what your ideal weight should be, often within a particular range. All these charts are based on height, with some having other divisions as well, including a breakdown by age or bone structure: the usual choices are small, medium or large. Overall, most charts are within a few pounds of one another either way, but they seldom agree completely. One doctor, as mentioned in *Folk Medicine* by D C Jarvis, has devised a system whereby (1) you measure your height (without shoes on); (2) multiply the number of inches over 5 feet by 5.5; (3) add the amount calculated from step (2) to 110. This is said to provide your ideal weight in pounds. If you happen to be less than 5 feet tall, then multiply the number of inches under 5 feet by 5.5 and subtract that amount from 110.

Slimming clubs fall short in one particular area: very little is learned about the health aspects of dieting; most focus solely on weight loss. While it is true that the amount of calories consumed is directly linked to weight gain or loss, the quality of those calories should also be considered. To say that it is OK to have a 'special treat' once in a while, particularly when calorie intake has been low, and then offering a list of relatively low-calorie biscuits and sweets, is really missing the mark, particularly if the items on the list tend to be of the non-nutritional sort. *Low-calorie does not necessarily mean healthy,* and this should be made clear. There really does need to be an emphasis shift to make the two aspects of diet go hand in hand. If the club is really concerned with the client's welfare, and not just their fee, they might consider including information on the health benefits (or otherwise) of recommended foods. An ideal slimming programme should encompass calorie control while encouraging better eating habits.

I would still recommend a slimming club if discipline is what you need to help shed those pounds. Alternatively, you might have several friends who also want to lose weight, in which case you can form your own weekly get-together, keeping track of one another's progress. Following the dietary advice given in Chapters 7 and 10, together with a weekly visit to a slimming club or group, may be just the right combination to get rid of excess weight permanently.

For further information about the nearest club in your area you can contact the head offices listed below, or check your local newspaper. Be aware, however, that advertisements frequently appear making claims about quick weight loss. These are often product-related and need to be checked out carefully.

For your nearest slimming club branch, contact the following organisations:

WelshSlim 30 High Street, Cowbridge, South Glamorgan CF7 7AG, telephone: (0446) 774141.

Slimming World (head office) Miles Paley Ltd, 34 High Street, South Normanton, Derbyshire DE55 2BP, telephone: (0773) 811247.

Weight Watchers UK (head office) Kidwells Park House, Kidwells Park Drive, Maidenhead, Berks SL6 8YT, telephone: (0628) 777077.

'WONDER DIETS' – A BRIEF LOOK AT A FEW

Every year sees at least one new diet discovery that claims to be the panacea to finally get those inches off and that weight down. Among the more sensible ones (others being referenced elsewhere in this book and in the Bibliography), is the hip and thigh diet created by Rosemary Conley. After her doctor told her that if she wanted to avoid surgery for gallstones she needed to go on a very low fat diet, she promptly complied. As a side benefit she lost inches, particularly in her hips and thighs, something that she claims she was unable to accomplish even when she lost weight in the past.

As a rule of thumb, Conley's hip and thigh diet stresses that any food which contains more than ½ oz/12 g fat per 4 oz/100 g should be avoided. This would automatically eliminate food products high in butter and oil. Fried food is out and only lean meat is acceptable.

In 1979 Dr Herman Tarnower took America by storm with the Scarsdale Diet. As the book cover of the fifth printing of *The Scarsdale Diet* in 1980 proclaimed, there were 21 printings in 1979. Menus are provided for a week's worth of meals. One of the rules is that you must eat only what is assigned. Although you do not have to eat everything listed, you cannot make substitutions or additions. Carrots and celery are the only things allowed for between-meal snacks.

Another of the ground rules is that 'you should not remain on the basic SMD (Scarsdale Medical Diet) for more than two weeks at a time'. A 'keep trim' diet is provided if more weight needs to be lost. This consists of lists of 'do's and 'don't's. It is further recommended that the SMD should be employed whenever excessive weight returns.

The Beverly Hills Diet provides a list of 'ten commandments' to provide a psychological edge: sensible sayings such as 'Set realistic goals. Don't set yourself up to fail. Don't be a victim' and 'You become a thin person . . . by letting go of the fat person – physically, intellectually and emotionally'. The diet itself spans five weeks with specific foods that must be eaten in a specific order. For example, the first week consists of eating *only* specified fruit. Pineapple, for example, which has enzymatic properties for burning off fat. In fact, on Day One of the diet, you can eat as much pineapple as you want followed by two bananas. The rules are strict and the allowable food choices are few.

The Doctor's Quick Weight Loss Diet, by Irwin Maxwell Stillman and Samm Sinclair Baker (presumably the same person who co-authored *The Complete Scarsdale Medical Diet* with Herman Tarnower), boasts about being able to lose 5 to 15 pounds a week with a safe new diet breakthrough. Again there are rigid rules allowing only certain foods to be eaten. These foods consist of: grilled, boiled, smoked or baked lean meat; skinless chicken and turkey; lean fish such as plaice, haddock, cod; shellfish such as shrimp, scallops, lobster, clams, crabs. Fish and meat can be either baked, grilled or boiled (horseradish and ketchup sauce is allowable in small amounts). Also allowed are: eggs cooked as you like them as long as no oil or other types of fat are used; cottage cheese or cheese made with skimmed milk; eight ½ pint/300 ml glasses of water daily or more if you like; coffee, tea, and non-caloric soda may be taken freely as long as no sugar, cream or milk is added. It is recommended that a daily dose of vitamin supplements accompany the diet — and no wonder as the diet is basically all protein.

MEAL REPLACEMENTS AND OTHER AIDS TO WEIGHT LOSS

There are quite a number of meal replacement plans available. Newspapers and magazines are cluttered with advertisements for them, and chemists and healthfood shops usually have an assortment on their shelves. The idea is to replace one or two meals a day with a powder you mix with milk; a solid bar; a sachet to dissolve in water (hot or cold as appropriate); a packet of biscuits, and suchlike. Various forms of hunger-suppressant tablets are also available. If they are chewed prior to mealtime they are supposed to suppress the appetite.

There is a range of other slimming techniques to choose from. A number of companies offer slimming videos and tapes. Through hypnosis, these provide subliminal suggestions that are supposed to 're-educate your subconscious mind'. Exercise tapes and videos are also available. Various kinds of exercise equipment can be found in shops and these include bikes and weights. Other special equipment is offered from a number of companies via mail order. These can be special high-tech machines in varying ranges, usually more in line with your wallet rather than your body type. There is even a postal slimming service. It is easy to find information on any of these options, should you desire to, from most women's magazines, especially, of course, from those dedicated to slimming.

And if all else fails there is always the diet pig, a plastic invention from the States which lives in the refrigerator and squeaks whenever the door is opened ...

It can all get very confusing. Some diets are made up almost entirely of protein while others have as little as possible. In many cases the menu plans can be very rigid and this makes dieting difficult, especially if you go out to work or have meals to prepare for others. Some of the ingredients that go into meal replacement plans may be questionable. For example, they all seem to have at least one form of sugar, with the majority having at least two different variations of sugar. In addition to the sugar, some also include the artificial sweetener aspartame.

The use of subliminal messages is something else that should be questioned. Exercise should be a part of every healthy lifestyle but it is important to know what you are doing or to have professional instruction. As for machine aids, they may be helpful but they should not be a substitute for calorie control when slimming. And, of course, there is always the question of what happens when, if you have been able to discipline yourself enough to stick with it without cheating and you actually lose the weight desired, you go back to your normal eating regime.

▶ GO TO ▶   ● *Maintain* healthy *loss, page 107*

14 Nutrients, vitamins and minerals

Ideally, your diet should contain all the necessary ingredients required to keep you healthy. These ingredients, of course, include an adequate supply of vitamins and minerals and these are discussed in the second part of this chapter.

Fats and proteins are the two main structural components that make up our bodies and carbohydrates supply the major source of energy. When you cut out or cut down on either it is important to understand the various options available and the benefits that they provide.

FATS AND FATTY ACIDS

Next to water, fat is the most abundant substance in our body. It assists the body to absorb vitamins A, D, E and K as these vitamins are soluble in fat rather than water. Fat is essential for the production of hormones and as a component of organs and cell walls. All fats are made up of triglycerides (one molecule of glycerine linked to three molecules of fatty acid).

Fatty acids are normally present in the bowel as by-products of the breakdown of certain foods; their role is to lubricate feces and help maintain the proper balance between bacteria and yeast. Certain fatty acids cannot be produced by the body and therefore it is essential that they are obtained from food sources.

There are three basic types of fats:

Saturated: these are usually solid at room temperature and are mainly of animal origin (beef, pork, lamb, poultry, butter, cream, eggs, lard, cheese) with the exception of coconut oil, and palm oil.

Monounsaturated fats: these are soft or liquid at room temperature but can solidify when cold. Sources include olive oil, nuts and some fruits.

Polyunsaturated fats: generally liquid or soft at both room and cooler temperatures. These are usually of vegetable origin except for certain fish oils such as mackerel, salmon, trout, sardines and herring, which are classified as Omega-3 essential fatty acids. Other polyunsaturated oils include safflower, sunflower, sesame, soya and corn, with some of these falling into the Omega-3 category as well.

Most fatty acids are produced in the body, as required, from carbohydrates. However, there are certain polyunsaturated fatty acids that cannot be produced by the body, hence the term 'essential fatty acids', which indicates that they must be obtained from food sources. Essential fatty acids are also sometimes known as vitamin F and they are vital for cell membranes, nerve fibres and brain cells among other things. Essential fatty acid food sources include fish oils and oily fish such as cod, mackerel, herring and salmon, and vegetable oils (see above).

Unfortunately, it seems that all polyunsaturates are not equal. According to Robert Erdmann and Meirion Jones in their book *Fats, Nutrition and Health,* there are two forms of polyunsaturates, known as *cis* and *trans.* The difference lies in their configuration. *Trans* fatty acids are a product of a number of food processing methods, particularly when enormous pressure and temperatures are used and this renders them unable to perform the life-giving functions in the body that *cis* polyunsaturates provide. The less processing an oil is subjected to, the better in this respect.

LECITHIN AND CHOLESTEROL

Fats also contain lecithin and cholesterol. Lecithin breaks up fats, keeping them liquid, and helps distribute them throughout the body. Lecithin is a component of bile and is stored in the gall bladder where it prevents cholesterol from hardening and forming gall stones. Lecithin also helps prevent cholesterol from being deposited in the arteries. In addition, lecithin is essential for healthy skin and nails. The best sources can be found in polyunsaturated oils and all soya products. Lecithin is also available from animal sources such as eggs, but because these sources contain saturated fats they are perhaps less desirable.

Cholesterol is made from fatty acids and asterol (a solid alcohol) and is wax-like in appearance. It is essential for life and is a component of all cells and is in fact manufactured by the body. In excess, however, it can be dangerous. Externally it is only found in animal products such as eggs, milk, butter, seafood and, of course, meat.

The absorption of cholesterol depends on a number of factors including the level of non-nutrient fibre in the diet. Fibre binds to cholesterol helping to eliminate it. As cholesterol does not dissolve in the blood, any excess is transported by special protein carriers known as lipoproteins. There are two types of lipoproteins, both produced in the liver and known as low-density and high-density lipoproteins. The high-density lipoproteins take the cholesterol to the liver, where it is broken down and eliminated. However, low-density lipoproteins take the cholesterol to the body tissues, which includes the blood vessel walls, where it is then deposited. Over time, these deposits can accumulate and cause the vessels to become narrower (see atherosclerosis, Chapter 4).

The levels of cholesterol in the blood are increased by the consumption of saturated fatty acids and a high level of body fat. Factors which can lower cholesterol include an increase in fibre intake, vitamin E, lecithin, calcium, magnesium and zinc and consumption of monosaturated and polyunsaturated fatty acids. However, it is felt that some polyunsaturated fatty acids will also reduce the beneficial high density lipoproteins. Monounsaturated fatty acids and essential fatty acids, such as Omega–3 found in fish oils, only reduces the harmful low density lipoproteins. Regular exercise is also helpful in lowering cholesterol.

There has been some disagreement recently about the benefit of polyunsaturated fats. When polyunsaturated fatty acids became popular, two factors were very important. Firstly, vitamin E was included. The benefit of the added vitamin E was that it protected against oxidation, thus protecting the oil or fat from becoming rancid from over-exposure to oxygen. Secondly, it was thought that polyunsaturated oils would be used cold as a dressing for salads, etc., not for frying. However, because they have come to be used as cooking oils, a problem arises: it seems that when heated to high temperatures, polyunsaturated oils react with oxygen to release free radicals which can be harmful to health and may be carcinogenic.

Another product that is not well understood is margarine. Most margarines are hydrogenated. Through the process of hydrogenation oil is transformed into a spreadable consistency. The advantage of doing this is mainly to benefit the manufacturer because it allows for longer shelf life. The processing, however, creates *trans* fatty acids.

Fats in summary
Daily dietary intake should ideally consist of no more than 25% fat. A good guideline would be to ensure that a higher percentage of polyunsaturated fat as opposed to saturated fat is consumed. Additionally, it is recommended that for cooking purposes cold pressed virgin olive oil is used as most other oils oxidise and turn rancid at high temperatures. Olive oil also provides more of the naturally occurring nutrients than the more highly processed alternatives. Keep oil in a cool dark place to avoid too much

interaction with light, which can cause the creation of free radicals (see Glossary of terms).

Sources of beneficial fatty acids include evening primrose oil, coconut oil, linseed oil, olive oil, spinach, kale, parsley, green pepper, salmon and mackerel.

CARBOHYDRATES

These are produced by plants and made up of the elements carbon, hydrogen and oxygen. Carbohydrates are an important source of energy for the body. Each gram provides approximately 4 kilocalories. Carbohydrates are broken down by the body into glucose and any excess is stored in the liver and muscles in the form of glycogen with extreme excesses being converted to stored fat.

Unrefined carbohydrates like wholewheat bread, brown rice, pasta, pulses, potatoes, vegetables (especially starchy root varieties) and fruits, are excellent choices for a healthy diet. Refined carbohydrates on the other hand are best avoided, from both slimming and health points of view. Refined carbohydrates include sugar-rich foods such as cakes, biscuits and processed cereals (cornflakes, for example).

Complex carbohydrates, on the other hand, are completely different in nature. *The old myth about carbohydrates being fattening, and therefore to be avoided when slimming, is not true.* It is necessary, however, to be particular about the choice of carbohydrates in the diet. Basically there are two kinds of carbohydrates: sugar and starch. Sugars, the so-called simple carbohydrates, are quickly absorbed into the bloodstream. Their effect does not last long and you often get a craving sensation which prompts the taking of additional sugar-drenched carbohydrates.

Starches, however, are complex carbohydrates and must be broken down into simple sugars by the body before they can be absorbed. Energy is released at a slow and steady rate. If the starches are high in fibre, the amount necessary to satisfy the appetite is less because of the added bulk that fibre provides.

Fibre
Fibre is found in the cell walls of plants. It passes through the body without being absorbed and fulfils a number of functions. It helps to prevent constipation and other bowel disorders, helps prevent gallstones, helps to keep blood cholesterol levels down (important in reducing the risk of heart disease), and provides a satisfying feeling of fullness without excessive calories. Foods rich in fibre include wholemeal bread, baked potatoes, brown rice, wholemeal pasta, raw vegetables and fresh fruit.

Carbohydrates in summary
A healthy diet should be made up mainly of unrefined fibre-rich carbohydrates because they are rich in starch with little simple sugar and they contain essential vitamins and minerals. One of the problems with refined carbohydrates is that as a result of the processing that takes place, much of the vitamins and minerals are lost. We end up eating empty calories. In addition, the fibre content is removed and this in itself can cause unnecessary overeating.

PROTEIN

The word protein comes from the Greek *proteios*, which means 'in the first place'. Protein is made up of one or more chains of amino acids and forms the structural material of muscles, tissues and organs. Amino acids are important in the manufacture of certain hormones and enzymes in addition to being essential in regulating functions of the body, including growth and maintenance. Protein is also important for the synthesis of antibodies produced by the immune system. Excess protein is converted by the body into glucose which can be used as an energy source. Because there are nine amino acids that cannot be produced by the body (leucine, isoleucine, lysine, methionine, phenylalanine, threonine, tryptophan, valine and histidine) it is essential that we get enough protein each day to meet these needs.

Although protein is obtained from both animals and vegetables, the precise make up of these proteins differs. The nine amino acids that are not produced by the human body are found in meat and fish and are therefore called 'complete proteins'; proteins from plant sources lack one or more of the essential amino acids, and so are called 'incomplete proteins'. Of course, by mixing various plant foods properly at mealtimes, meals providing complete proteins can easily be created (see Table 7). It is important that

---

Table 7: Complementary vegetable proteins

When eaten at the same meal, the following food combinations will provide all of the essential amino acids (complete protein) without the use of meat or dairy products.

corn or wheat with beans

rice or millet with peas, beans or lentils

nuts or seeds with pulses

soya beans are complete proteins (although they are somewhat low in the amino acid methionine)

---

this balancing of foods to form complete proteins be accomplished at each meal, otherwise some of the protein consumed may not be properly utilised.

One of the major arguments made against alternative diets, particularly the vegan diet, is that they do not allow for adequate protein. School children are given their daily bottle of milk and we are taught that the best sources of protein are meat and dairy products. Indeed, the four basic food groups taught in school, and commonly accepted as gospel, are: vegetable/fruit, bread/cereal, milk (including cheese) and meat. Most parents usually do want to provide 'what is best' for their children. Because of early experiments done on rats which showed faster growth as a result of animal protein as opposed to plant protein, it was assumed that animal protein was 'better'. It is interesting to note that the percentage of protein in human milk is 5% as opposed to 49% in milk from rats. Also it normally takes about 180 days for a human baby to double its birth weight as opposed to four days for a baby rat. We can pretty safely assume from this data that not only do baby rats require more protein than human babies, but they also grow faster.

Unfortunately, a lot more has been assumed and special interest groups like dairy and meat industries have been quick to pick up on the animal protein mythology. Although it is true that a complete protein can be obtained from a single animal source, by proper food combining (Table 7) the same results can be achieved — and without the added saturated fat that comes along with the animal protein which has been shown to be a leading cause of so many of our modern diseases.

Additionally, research seems to indicate now that we do not need as much protein as was once thought. Many nutritionists believe that no more than 10% of total calorie intake should consist of protein and that it would be difficult not to meet these requirements, even on a vegetarian or vegan diet. Nathan Pritikin, considered by many in America to be the foremost expert on nutrition, thought that only 6% of total caloric intake need consist of protein (his diet programme, strangely enough, recommends between 10 and 15% protein). As human milk, required at the most intensive growth period of life, contains only 5%

protein, it would seem Pritikin's assessment of human needs comes closest to that decided by nature itself.

It is also felt that excessive protein can put a strain on the kidneys in addition to increasing body fat (remember unused protein can be turned into glucose which, if not used, can be stored as fat). Excessive protein can also cause B3 (niacin) and B6 deficiencies and cause a loss of calcium, which will have a weakening effect on bones (see osteoporosis, Chapter 4).

As Frances Lappé pointed out in her much-acclaimed book *Diet for a Small Planet:* 'Virtually all traditional societies based their diets on protein complementarity; they used grain and legume (pulse) combinations as their main source of protein and energy . . .'

FOOD COMBINING

Other aspects of food combining are also important. The time it takes to digest a meal depends on the consistency and composition of the food eaten. The quantity eaten will also have an effect. It only takes between 15 minutes to half an hour for liquids to leave the stomach. Fats have a tendency to slow down the secretion of the gastric juices needed for digestion, which means they take longer to digest. Proteins and carbohydrates are somewhere in between, with carbohydrates being quickest of all to digest.

Different foods require different digestive enzymes. If an assortment of foods from different categories are eaten at once, not all may be fully digested. (See Chapter 15 where an outline of the Hay diet is given).

VITAMINS AND MINERALS

A vitamin is any of a group of substances that cannot be synthesised by the body but is required, in very small amounts, for healthy growth and maintenance. They are divided into two groups: A, D, E and K, which are fat-soluble – dependent on the presence of fat, minerals, other fat-soluble vitamins and bile for proper utilisation and absorption; and B-complex and C, which are water-soluble – broken down by water allowing any excess to be eliminated.

Although potential visual symptoms associated with deficiency are described below under some of the vitamin categories, self diagnosis and therapy is not advised. A qualified therapist should be consulted and dietary supplementation recommended if required. It is possible that other symptoms such as headaches, sore eyes, etc. may be the cause of a deficiency in one or more nutrients. Taking too much of one vitamin may cause a deficiency in another. A deficiency in one vitamin may have an effect on other nutrients as well. It is essential to obtain qualified medical assistance to determine the cause of the problem. Certainly nutrient deficiency should be a consideration and appropriate testing should be carried out. Individual needs differ and so any recommended daily amounts must be considered as guideline information only.

Vitamin A and beta carotene

Vitamin A is synthesised in the body from carotene, which is found in many fruits and vegetables. In an already synthesised form, vitamin A (retinol) is found in foods derived from animal sources (milk, cheese, etc.) and in liver because, as with humans, that is where vitamin A is stored. Vitamin A has the following properties:

• stimulates and enhances immune system function;
• is important for bone growth;
• aids in growth, development and maintenance of epithelial cells (skin cells);
• protects cells against infection by assisting in the production of mucus.

A strong indication that beta carotene can protect against the presence of carcinogens was shown as a result of a 19-year-study conducted by Richard B. Shekelle (*Lancet*, November 1981).

Symptoms which can point to a lack of vitamin A include a reduction in the moistness of the eyes, inability to adjust properly from dim to bright light (as in night blindness) and brittle nails that break easily. Follicular keratosis, which is a particular kind of roughness of the skin, can also be caused by lack of vitamin A.

It is important to remember that because vitamin A is fat-soluble it does not get broken down in water for excretion and if taken in excess over long periods of time it can cause toxicity. Being fat-soluble also means that cooking will not destroy any of the vitamin and in fact puréeing or mashing may allow for easier absorption. Juicing is another method which makes the carotene more easily absorbed.

Carotenes: all green leafy vegetables and yellow fruits and vegetables, carrots, sweet potatoes, yams, apricots, cantaloupe melons, broccoli, squash, yellow corn, palm oil, spinach, turnip greens, kale, tomatoes, mangoes, papayas, peaches, nectarines, pumpkin.

Retinol: fish, especially halibut, shark, cod, salmon, herring, sardines; liver, butter, cheese, eggs, milk.

Vitamin B-complex
Vitamin B-complex is actually a group of 12 vitamins which are similar to each other and primarily function as co-enzymes to help maintain a proper rate of metabolism. They also help in the creation of red blood cells and assist in the maintenance of healthy organs, nervous system, hair and skin. Because they are closely related it is necessary that a balanced ration be available in the body to ensure optimal efficiency. A shortage of one can cause impairment to the function of the other B vitamins.

B vitamins are sensitive to heat and light, so if possible it is best to eat the food sources raw or lightly steamed. A large percentage of B vitamins are lost when foods are processed. This includes canning and preserving.

Vitamin B1 (thiamin) – co-enzyme in carbohydrate metabolism. Also important to ensure proper nerve function. A factor in the production of RNA. Helps keep the heart muscle resilient. (SOURCES: wholegrain cereals, beans, meat, potatoes, nuts, sunflower seeds, peanuts, wheatgerm, fish, eggs, green vegetables, apples.)

Vitamin B2 (riboflavin) – important for growth and maintenance of tissue. Helps in the breakdown of carbohydrates, fats and proteins. Helpful for the nervous system and in iron assimilation. Works with vitamin A in maintaining proper vision. Maintains healthy red blood cells, skin and eyes. (SOURCES: liver, milk, yoghurt, cheese, eggs, yeast. Moderate amounts are also found in spinach, fish, oatmeal, cauliflower, cabbage, carrots, potatoes, wholemeal bread.)

Vitamin B3 (niacin) – promotes healthy skin, and is helpful for the nervous system and digestive tract. It can have a positive effect on cholesterol levels. Helps control the release of energy from carbohydrates. Niacin can be formed in the body from the essential amino acid tryptophan. (SOURCES: meat, fish, poultry, peanut butter, wholegrain bread, cereals, yeast, brown rice, beans, oatmeal, dried fruit.)

Pantothenic acid (B5) – aids in releasing energy from fats and carbohydrates. Helps to utilise other vitamins. Takes part in the synthesis of cholesterol and fatty acids. Aids adrenal glands in the production of essential hormones. Protects against cellular damage due to radiation exposure. Important to the immune system. Sometimes considered to be an anti-stress vitamin. It is highly distributed in foods from animal sources, whole grains, legumes (pulses) and to a lesser extent in fruits and vegetables.

Vitamin B6 (pyridoxine) – helps regulate the use of carbohydrates, fats and proteins and assists in red blood cell maintenance. Helps to reconstitute amino acids derived from food protein. Important for immune system maintenance. Helps to keep sodium/potassium levels in balance. Important to the nervous system. Works with magnesium to prevent the occurence of kidney stones; decreases stiffness/numbness resulting from arthritis. Deficiency can result in dry itchy skin and cracks at the corner of the mouth. (SOURCES: meat, soya beans, broad beans, bananas, pears, whole grains, salmon, herring, green vegetables.)

Vitamin B12 (cyanocobalamin) – necessary for the synthesis of nucleic acids and bone marrow; responsible for maintenance of myelin in the nervous system and aids in the proper functioning of folic acid (another of the B complex, see below). Needed to make red blood cells. Helps stabilise body weight and convert food into energy. Deficiency is very rare except possibly when a strict vegan diet is followed; deficiency will affect nearly all body tissues and have a degenerating effect on the nervous system. (SOURCES: liver, fish, shellfish, milk, cheese, eggs. NOTE: fermented foods such as soy sauce and tempeh contain some vitamin B12.)

Choline – important in the synthesis of lecithin and involved in the transport of fat in the body. Helps prevent fatty deposits in the liver. Helps to inhibit formation of gall stones. Assists nervous system by helping to maintain a strong myelin sheath. (SOURCES: wheatgerm, bran, lecithin, soya beans.)

Inositol – helps the liver to handle fats and aids in the production of lecithin by the body. Helps to prevent fatty deposits in arteries. Although it is classified as a vitamin, it can be synthesised. It is, however, found in many food sources, particularly in bran.

Biotin – essential for the metabolism of fat and is involved in fatty acid synthesis. Helps regulate carbohydrate metabolism. Deficiency is rare. (SOURCES: fresh vegetables, milk, meat, eggs, cheese, rice, nuts.)

Folic acid – important in the synthesis of nucleic acids and works with vitamin B_{12}. It is important for cell reproduction within the fetus. Stimulates the production of hydrochloric acid needed for digestion. Helps nervous system. (SOURCES: liver, green leafy vegetables, nuts, legumes [pulses], fish, wholemeal bread, bananas, meat, eggs.)

PABA (Para-aminobenzoic acid) – helps make proteins and blood cells. Important for healthy hair and healthy intestines. Used in suntan oils because of its sunscreen capability. The body can produce PABA in the intestines. (SOURCES: liver, yeast, wheatgerm, molasses.)

Vitamin B-complex deficiency has been linked with mental illness because these vitamins are an important component in the production of neurotransmitters, the chemical substances that the brain uses to send messages. Another contributor to vitamin B deficiency, especially thiamine (B_1), is refined carbohydrates. Beri beri, for example, a disease caused by a lack of thiamin, did not become a problem until people started eating white rice and white flour. This is because the two parts of the grain which contain the thiamin, the bran and the scutellum (the thin layer separating the starchy part from the germ), are lost during the 'refining' process.

Obvious symptoms that may be caused by a lack of vitamin B-complex include ridges on the tongue or a dark blueish coloured tongue, skin rash, mouth sores, or cracks appearing in the corner of the mouth. Vitamin B_2 deficiency may also cause oily skin and hair loss.

(SOURCES FOR VITAMIN B-COMPLEX: brewer's yeast, liver [but

see Chapter 18], whole grains, beans, leafy green vegetables, carrots, salmon, carob, wheatgerm, rice bran, eggs,
sunflower seeds.)

Vitamin C (ascorbic acid)

Vitamin C is a multi-purpose vitamin which is involved in
most of the body's biochemical reactions. Being water-
soluble, vitamin C is not stored in the body and must be
replenished daily. Cooking should be minimal, preferably
using the steaming method to minimise loss of vitamin C to
the cooking water. Much of the value of nutrients such as
vitamin C will be lost in canned, frozen or processed food
although those foods may have once had an abundant
supply.

Linus Pauling, PhD, winner of two Nobel Prizes, has done
much research on vitamin C and feels that the most important aspect of it is its ability to stimulate the immune system, thus enabling the body to fight off viral and bacterial
invaders. Pauling, in his book *Vitamin C and the Common
Cold*, makes the case of vitamin C as a preventative agent
against the common cold. Although this caused much controversy at the time, and there is still debate over the large
doses he advocated, it is now pretty much accepted that
vitamin C does play a role in combating colds.

Vitamin C is also involved in the following processes:

• protects cells against damage from oxidation;
• defends against disease-causing microbes;
• is essential for healthy bones, teeth and blood vessels;
• aids in the production of collagen, a protein that is the
principal material of fibrous connective tissue found in
tendons, skin, bone, cartilage and ligaments;
• stimulates the body's production of interferon (a protein
which is produced by cells infected with a virus and has the
ability to inhibit that viral growth);
• assists with the healing of wounds;

• aids in the prevention of blood clots;
• has antihistamine properties that are useful in combating many allergens;
• helps in cholesterol maintenance by aiding in the process which converts it to bile acids, allowing it to be eliminated from the body;
• combats stress by promoting calmness and mental tranquillity;
• is antibacterial – helps white blood cells in destroying invading bacteria;
• has been shown to be helpful in both the prevention and treatment of cancer as detailed in *Cancer and Vitamin C*, by Ewan Cameron and Linus Pauling, which is based on a five-year trial conducted in Scotland in the 1970s;
• works to reduce the potency of, and help eliminate, toxins in the body, including nitrates (from food preservatives), pesticide residues in food, cadmium, lead, mercury, arsenic, benzene and carbon monoxide;
• aids in mental health.

Deficiency of vitamin C can cause scurvy, which is characterised by sore, swollen and bleeding gums, loose teeth and anaemia. Vitamin C can also be leached from the body as a result of drugs, smoking, alcohol and caffeine.

(SOURCES: citrus fruits, green vegetables such as broccoli, green pepper, cabbage, spinach, carrots, bananas, peas, lettuce, apples, plums, Brussels sprouts, as well as cauliflower, tomatoes, cantaloupe, strawberries, kiwi fruit, pineapple, potatoes with skin, alfalfa, sprouts (mung beans, lentils and sunflower seeds) and cayenne pepper.

Bioflavonoids
These substances are found in the white membrane and between the sections of citrus fruits. They also come from the skin of apricots, cherries, grapes, plums and blackberries. They protect vitamin C from being destroyed by oxidation.

The benefits derived from bioflavonoids include strengthening of blood vessels, promotion of healing and helping prevent high blood pressure.

Vitamin D (cholecalciferol)

Probably the best source is produced in the body as a result of the action of sunlight through the skin. Vitamin D stimulates the absorption of calcium from the intestines and helps to regulate calcium and phosphorous levels in the blood. It also helps in the maintenance of bones and teeth.

Vitamin D deficiency results in rickets in children where bones are malformed and do not harden. In adults the disease is known as osteomalacia, where the bones lose calcium, replacing the normally hard substance with softer tissue. Since vitamin D is fat-soluble, excess can be stored in the body and can cause toxicity. (SOURCES: milk, eggs, liver, fish oils, herring, salmon, mackerel, sardines, cheese, butter.)

Vitamin E (tocopherol)

Dr Wilfred Shute, a leading researcher on vitamin E in the States, is convinced that there is a direct correlation between the vitamin and heart disease. For example, coronary thrombosis, a condition where a blood clot partially or fully blocks one of the arteries which leads to the heart, was not known prior to this century. Coincidentally, some may say, it was in 1900 when new techniques in milling were introduced and a main source of vitamin E, the germ of wheat, was no longer part of the daily bread. Taking this as a clue, Dr Wilfred Shute and his brother, Dr Evan Shute, gave vitamin E therapy to heart patients. They found that those taking extra vitamin E had more rapid and complete recoveries. Yet another benefit of vitamin E is that it regulates blood clotting, breaking up clots without disturbing normal clotting functions such as wound healing. It ensures that blood platelets, which are necessary for clotting, are available but also helps to prevent new, unnecessary clots from forming.

Vitamin E also has the following properties:

• helps to lower levels of cholesterol in the blood;
• is necessary for the effective use of oxygen in the blood, ensuring that organs get adequate supplies;
• keeps blood vessels open and helps strengthen the walls of both capillaries and red blood cells;
• helps to strengthen the immune system;
• helps maintain the function and structure of the human nervous system;
• helps in the treatment of burns by bringing oxygen and nutrients to the affected area as well as curtailing the development of bacteria;
• helps protect cells and rid the body of free radicals (works in conjunction with selenium) and carcinogens;
• can help reduce fatigue;
• has an antioxidant property which protects unsaturated fatty acids from becoming rancid.

Although vitamin E is fat-soluble, toxicity from any excess in the diet does not seem to be a problem. Deficiency is mainly due to diets which favour processed foods at the expense of fresh vegetables and whole grains. The germ (where vitamin E is found) is removed from the wheat when white flour is produced. Even so-called 'enriched' bread is lacking in vitamin E. Bread may be called enriched because some, but not all, of the B vitamins that were originally part of the grain before processing removed them are replaced. One might ask, why take them out in the first place? The loss of vitamin E in processing also happens in the case of vegetable oils unless they are cold pressed.

If you are considering using a supplement, *it is important to know that natural vitamin E is almost twice as effective as synthetic vitamin E.* In its natural form, vitamin E is identified as 'd-alpha tocopherol' whereas the synthetic version is known as 'dl-alpha tocopherol'. A subtle difference in chemistry that really counts.

(SOURCES: wheatgerm is the richest source. Other sources include whole grains, nuts, whole eggs, polyunsaturated vegetable oils [cold pressed only], leafy vegetables, sunflower seeds, seaweed, peanuts, soya beans, liver [but see Chapter 18], sprouts.)

Vitamin K

Vitamin K is necessary for the synthesis of urinary glycoprotein, which inhibits calcium oxalate crystalline growth resulting in kidney stones. It is also important in blood clotting.

Vitamin K is produced by the body in the intestines and so deficiency is very unlikely.

(SOURCES: green leafy vegetables, cauliflower, sprouts, peas, broccoli, fish oils, liver.)

MINERALS

Minerals are inorganic substances obtained from the earth. A number of them play an essential role for developing and maintaining a healthy body.

A list of food sources for each mineral is given at the end of each section below. A particular mineral may appear in other sources as well, but I have endeavoured to mention those foods that contain the best sources.

Calcium

Calcium is of vital importance to the body as it is the major component of bones and teeth. The bones also store excess calcium which can then be used for other body functions as required. Calcium has the following properties:

- essential for nerve function;
- essential for muscle contraction;

- important as a component in blood and for blood clotting;
- able to modulate hormones and enzymes.

The parathyroid glands actually regulate the amount of calcium in the blood and this is normally kept at a consistent level. A drop in calcium levels can result in muscle cramps.

For proper absorption, calcium needs vitamin D and protein (although *an excess* of protein along with other factors may contribute to calcium loss and this can result in a weakening and thinning of bones – see osteoporosis, Chapter 4). Proper exercise also promotes calcium absorption. (SOURCES: milk, cheese, yoghurt, eggs, butter, fish bones [i.e. sardines, whitebait and canned salmon], tofu, green leafy vegetables [particularly cabbage, kale and broccoli], ice cream [especially dairy ice cream], sesame seeds, turnip, fruits.)

Some vegetables contain oxalic acid, which binds with calcium and so prevents the absorption of the calcium that is contained within that vegetable. These vegetables include: asparagus, beet greens, dandelion, parsley, sorrel and spinach. This does not mean that these vegetables should not be eaten, but you should not rely on them as a source of calcium. Oxalic acid is helpful to the gall bladder and kidneys.

Iron

Iron is an essential nutrient and the second most abundant metal, after aluminium, in the earth's crust. Iron is a component of haemoglobin (the pigment of red blood cells). Haemoglobin carries oxygen from the lungs to the tissues of the body for metabolic processes. Haemoglobin deficiency (lack of iron) causes anaemia, which reduces the efficiency of most of the body's functions.

It is also a component in myoglobin (found in red muscles) and cytochromes (protein pigments which function as respiratory enzymes). It seems that iron is only absorbed by the body as and when it is needed and this makes an overdose virtually impossible. Deficiency, however, is quite possible and, as mentioned above, the main cause of anaemia is iron deficiency. A lack of iron can also impair the immune system.

(SOURCES: liver [but see Chapter 18], curry powder, cocoa powder, molasses, cockles, oysters, winkles, meat, poultry, eggs, sardines, herring, salmon, haddock, parsley, cabbage, potatoes, dates, prunes, dried apricots, melon, blackberries, oatmeal, wholemeal flour, soya beans.) It should be noted that if iron pots are used for cooking, food will pick up additional iron as a result.

Magnesium

Magnesium is essential to the metabolic processes which convert food into energy. It helps to keep excess calcium away from soft tissues and is important for relaxing muscle function and helps prevent muscle cramps (it works in conjunction with calcium, which is needed to contract muscles).

High levels of toxic metals including lead, cadmium, mercury and aluminium can disturb the body's calcium-magnesium balance and this can result in calcium accumulation in the cells. (SOURCES: green vegetables, meat, fish, seafood, whole grains.)

Potassium

This is found mainly in the cells and helps maintain the body's internal environment and fluid balance. Potassium has the following properties:

- it is helpful to nerve impulse transmission;
- it stimulates movement of the intestinal tract.

Potassium loss can result from severe injury or any condition which results in a breakdown of cellular proteins.

Prolonged diarrhoea can also lead to potassium depletion. Excess potassium is excreted by the kidneys and so an overdose is unlikely.

(SOURCES: fresh fruit, especially bananas, grapes and plums, vegetables, dried fruit, nuts, whole grains, fish, poultry, beans, soya, molasses, cocoa, paprika, apple cider vinegar and honey mixture, cranberry juice, kelp.)

Phosphorus

This mineral is important to the basic biochemical mechanism (obtaining of energy) and is an essential component of blood and certain enzymes and hormones which control body functions. It works with calcium to strengthen bone.

In excess, however, phosphorus causes calcium to be leached from the bones. It can also neutralize the benefits from magnesium, manganese, zinc and copper and this in turn can lead to deficiences of these minerals.

(SOURCES: phosphorus is found in all living things – raw foods, wheatgerm, yeast, bran, beef, and also soft drinks, preserved foods, dairy substitutes.)

Selenium

There has been much debate over whether or not selenium is an important factor for cancer prevention because of its ability to neutralise free radicals. It has the following properties:

• aids in liver function;
• improves immune system response;
• protects against cadmium, mercury and other toxic minerals;
• is important for healthy hair, skin and eyes.

Selenium deficiency can impair the formation of antibodies, especially if vitamin E is also deficient. (SOURCES: meat, tuna fish, shellfish, whole grains, dairy products, onion, garlic, fruit, vegetables, especially broccoli and asparagus, tomatoes, mushrooms and Brazil nuts.)

Sodium (salt)

In a normal healthy diet enough salt is contained in the foods eaten so it is not actually necessary to add more. In association with potassium it helps in maintaining fluid balance in the body.

Excessive salt intake can result in hypertension (high blood pressure) which can then lead to other illnesses (see hypertension, Chapter 4). Salt also leaches calcium from the bones.

Salt deficiency, which causes muscular cramps, can result from excessively heavy perspiration or prolonged diarrhoea.

Zinc

Zinc has the following properties:

- essential for a properly functioning immune system;
- essential for tissue growth;
- important for skin maintenance, collagen production; helpful in the healing of wounds;
- helpful, along with vitamin C, in lowering the levels of lead in the blood;
- important to the formation of keratin which is a major component of hair;
- helpful in counteracting depression.

An obvious symptom of a potential zinc deficiency can be the appearance of white spots on the nails. Hair follicles are also affected, causing hair to fall out easily.

Fruits and vegetables are poor sources of zinc, and the phytic acid present in grains binds zinc and hinders the absorption, thus making grain products a source not to be relied on too heavily. (SOURCES: meat, liver [but see Chapter 18], milk, cheese, poultry, eggs, sardines, crab, oysters, pilchards, herring, beans, pumpkin seeds, mustard, soya beans, berries, peas.)

Other minerals needed in small amounts

Chromium – enables insulin to properly function. (SOURCES: yeast, beer, wholegrain cereals and breads, meat, cheese.)

Copper – together with iron, forms haemoglobin in the red blood cells. It works to release energy from food. (SOURCES: shellfish, meat, nuts, pulses, wholegrain cereals.)

Iodine – used mainly by the thyroid gland where the hormones it produces control the rate of body metabolism. (SOURCES: seafood, vegetables, milk, cereals.)

Manganese – functions to keep calcium out of arterial cells. (SOURCES: nuts, whole grains, green leafy vegetables.)

▶ GO TO ▶   ♦ *Vegetarian and* 'alternative' *diets, page 181.*

15 *Vegetarian and 'alternative' diets*

Most of us were brought up to believe that meat was a mandatory part of our daily diet because the protein it provided was necessary for our good health. However, abstinence from meat and animal by-products is by no means something new and unique to a 'fringe' lifestyle. Indeed, civilisations have survived on a meatless diet for thousands of years. Vegetarianism was the basis for a number of religious diets including Hinduism and Jainism. Diet was, and in some cases still is, an important aspect of religious life. A quick look back at a few of the ancient notions about food points up what many of us consider to be very modern concepts.

Meat taboos in India were based on the idea that many more people could be fed on grain crops as opposed to the meat from animals that grazed on the same amount of land (see Chapter 18). Early translations of the Bible suggest that the meaning of 'not eating of the forbidden fruit' had to do with unhealthy food. The Judaic religion forbids the eating of pork. It is known that it is not healthy to eat pork, particularly in hot climates. There are those today who feel that the parasites from pork are not killed no matter how long the meat is cooked. Cows were sacred in many religions and it was not until 1856 and at the request of the first American Ambassador to Japan that a cow was slaughtered in that country. Certain Hindu and Buddhist sects do not eat meat because they believe in reincarnation, and that the soul of an animal once resided in a human being.

Meat is a complete protein, which means that it contains all of the essential amino acids that are not produced in the body but are required by it. What we sometimes forget is that the complete protein found in the meat comes from the food the animal eats: *those essential amino acids are not naturally occurring in animals' bodies either.* By proper food combining, meals can easily contain the complete protein required without meat being part of the equation (see Table 7, page 163). A number of meatless diets are outlined below.

MACROBIOTIC DIET

The macrobiotic diet is based on the principle of achieving the perfect balance between yin and yang, the Eastern system of harmony. Yin or 'shade' is representative of the feminine principle, which is associated with dark, cold, yielding and negative force. Yang or 'sunlight' represents the male principle and is associated with light, heat, strength and positive force. The theory for this diet is that too much or too little of either of these opposites can produce an imbalance in the body which leads to illness.

Most foods can be categorised as yin or yang. Yin foods consist mainly of vegetables and fruits while yang foods consist of meat, fish and salty things. Brown rice and other cooked cereals are a combination of both yin and yang and are therefore considered to be balanced.

The ideal macrobiotic diet is considered to be organic grains with cooked vegetables and seeds, with occasional organic fruit. Foods containing sugar or additives are avoided. As meat and fish are very rarely eaten, the yang element is supplied by the use of salt, particularly sesame salt, and carbon, which is produced by slightly burning the grains.

Rice tends to be the key ingredient of this diet. It is both low in calories and expands in the stomach to provide a sense of fullness which lasts. This is because rice takes longer to digest than bread, the flour of which has been ground down due to the milling process. Rice also contains most of the essential amino acids required by the body from outside sources and complemented by pulses, will provide complete protein (page 163).

However, it has to be said that the macrobiotic diet is not an easy one to follow and it can lead to certain vitamin and mineral deficiencies.

FROM VEGAN TO VEGETARIAN, WITH A FEW VARIATIONS

The meatless diets that follow are listed in order from most to least restrictive. This means that all of the nutritional information provided in the discussion of the vegan diet will be appropriate for the vegetarian, and white meat vegetarian as well. Additional nutritional information given for the vegetarian will also be appropriate for the white meat vegetarian diet.

Vegan diet

The vegan diet excludes all products made from animal sources. This includes meat, fish, poultry, eggs, cheese, animal milk, honey and, of course, anything which includes one or more of these products as ingredients.

A number of studies have shown that a balanced vegan diet is low in saturated fat and refined sugar and high in fibre and polyunsaturated fat, a key factor in the prevention of degenerative disease.

The initial reaction to a vegan diet is that there is so little 'allowable' food to choose from. A closer look reveals the fallacy of that idea. Foods acceptable to the vegan diet include: fruits, vegetables, cereals, pulses, nuts, whole grains, soya milk, tofu, vegetable margarine and oils, sugar-free preserves and juices, and dried fruits. There are even a growing number of 'convenience foods' available that are suitable for vegans.

Despite some claims to the contrary, eating a vegan diet can provide all of the nutrients required for a healthy body. A good source of protein in a vegan diet comes from soya beans because they contain all of the essential amino acids (although they are low in methionine, see page 193). Other protein sources are: grains (rice, wheat, millet, oatmeal, rye); pulses (lentils, beans, peas); nuts (almonds, cashews, pecans, walnuts); and seeds (sesame, sunflower, etc). Sprouts and vegetables also contain some protein. The optimum protein potential is best obtained from proper food combining.

The sources for fats in a vegan diet are cereals, nuts, seeds, vegetable oils and margarine. Carbohydrate sources are grains, bread, pasta, cereals, pulses, nuts and certain vegetables. As they are usually unrefined, they also contain other essential nutrients. Cereals and pulses supply B vitamins, minerals and fibre.

General vitamin information is given in Chapter 14. Vegans can note specifically that vitamin A, while not occurring naturally in plant foods, can be made by the body from carotene, which comes from carrots, tomatoes, apricots, spinach, green vegetables and beansprouts. Foods acceptable to vegans that provide vitamin C include: citrus fruits, green vegetables, potatoes, beansprouts, tomatoes and berries. Although the best source of Vitamin D is from sunlight, it is also available from fortified margarine and fortified soya milk. Vitamin E is obtained from wheatgerm, beansprouts, polyunsaturated vegetable oils, nuts, pulses and some fruits and vegetables. Vitamin K is obtained from green vegetables, grains, kelp, alfalfa sprouts, spinach and soya oil.

It should be noted that although the primary sources of vitamin B12 are meat and dairy products, the vitamin is also found in seaweed, alfalfa, miso, tempeh (see Chapter 16), naturally-fermented soy sauce, kelp and many vegetables. In addition, soya milk and yeast extracts fortified with vitamin B12 can be obtained.

All the necessary mineral requirements of the body can be obtained from plant foods, including calcium which is available in nuts, soya products, dried fruits, beansprouts, pulses, seeds, grains and vegetables. For further information about veganism or the vegan diet contact: The Vegan Society Ltd., 7 Battle Road, St Leonards-on-Sea, East Sussex TN37 7AA.

Vegetarian diet

The reasons why vegetarians do not eat meat can vary. Some completely abhor the slaughter of animals, while others are more concerned about the potential health risk of eating animals treated with hormones and chemicals which are used to stimulate growth and mask disease. Again, the relatively high cost of meat has influenced some to increase the number of meatless meals they prepare each week – there are probably a large number of such 'part-time' vegetarians. There are also very sound ecological reasons for greatly reducing, if not completely eliminating, meat farming (see Chapter 18).

The use of dairy products and eggs distinguishes this form of diet from that of the vegan. Because these products are allowed, the term 'ovo-lacto vegetarian' is more descriptive and sometimes used. However, although many still use cow's milk, a growing number of vegetarians are switching to soya milk.

White meat and vegetarian diet

Some people stretch the term vegetarian to allow the occasional meal which includes fish or poultry. Strictly speaking, they are not vegetarians since the term implies a non-carnivore.

OTHER ALTERNATIVE DIETS

The Hay diet

The principle of this diet is food combination. Basically, to enhance digestion, proteins or acid fruits should not be eaten at the same meal with carbohydrates because they require different digestive processes. High protein foods (meat, cheese, eggs) require acid for the purposes of digestion, while carbohydrates need an alkaline milieu. The various enzymes necessary for the different processes may conflict with one another, resulting in less than perfect digestion. Dr Hay felt that each meal should be restricted to a particular food group thus optimising food digestion.

Foods for a protein meal include fresh meats, fish, poultry, cheese, eggs and nuts. These foods may be accompanied by acid fruits (grapefruit, orange, apple, apricot, prunes, cherries) and green vegetables (carrots and other root vegetables are also acceptable for combination). Potatoes should not be included in the protein meal. A salad consisting of one or a combination of lettuce, cabbage, celery, cress, tomatoes and peppers is suggested.

A starch-based meal could contain any of the following: cereals, brown rice, oatmeal, bread or pasta. These can be eaten with sweets, preferably made from natural sources like honey, dates and figs. Vegetables can include potato and salads but exclude tomatoes.

Food choices for the alkaline meal can consist of yoghurt or milk eaten with any green or root vegetable and any acid fruit (see above). Certain foods should also be avoided: vinegar, pickles, hot spices, foods that contain sugar, dried beans, chestnuts and rhubarb.

▶ GO TO ▶   ♦ *Food safety, page 199*

16 Healthy foods – where to find them

When I became a vegetarian, almost 10 years ago, I learned how to be a creative cook. Cookbooks for vegetarians were almost non-existent and little information was available on substitutions for ingredients that I wanted to avoid. Today there is an abundance of wonderful vegetarian cookbooks. In addition, there are many products – for example, textured vegetable protein – that offer the same benefits of what many would consider more questionable food sources. Vegetarian cooking has become exciting and in many ways more flexible than the standard meat-and-vegetable formula that so many of us grew up with.

This chapter contains information on what is generally thought of as 'fringe' foods. These food sources are becoming more and more popular, however, and are readily obtainable from any good healthfood shop. A growing number of food stores, including most of the large chains, are now stocking many of these items and will include more if they know the demand is there.

Agar agar

This is a gelatine substitute made from a sea vegetable. It contains protein, iodine and iron. Although it is also available in flakes and strips, it is easiest to use powdered. It is a good idea to check the label before purchasing to ensure that a sweetener or flavouring has not been added.

Bulgur wheat

This is cracked wheat which has been pre-cooked. It is a

staple grain of Eastern Europe and is used in the Middle
East as well. A typical bulgur wheat-based dish is tabouli.
To make it you need 4 oz/100 g bulgur wheat, juice of 1
lemon, 5 spring onions finely chopped, finely chopped parsley, 3 fl oz/100 ml apple cider vinegar, 3 fl oz/100 ml
tamari, 1 clove garlic, finely chopped, ¼ t ground pepper, 2
small diced tomatoes, 1 diced green pepper. Serve with
fresh mint. Pour boiling water over the bulgur to cover
wheat and let it sit. Blend the remaining ingredients, except
the tomatoes and pepper, together. When the bulgur is
ready (about 30 minutes – once water is absorbed), stir in
the mixture of ingredients and add the tomatoes and pepper.

Carob
Carob, a member of the legume family and sometimes
known as St John's bread, is a fleshy pod from an evergreen
tree which grows in the Middle East. It makes a healthy and
delicious alternative to chocolate. Although carob has 46%
natural sugar compared with cocoa, which has only 5.5%,
carob has 40% fewer calories. It is high in calcium and
potassium, contains no caffeine, and has less phosphorus
than cocoa. And, if that isn't enough to make you switch to
carob immediately, it is also low in fat, contains vitamins
B1, B3 and A, and is rich in protein and (as has been mentioned above) natural carbohydrates.

   Carob comes in block, chip, powder or syrup form and can
be purchased from any health shop and some groceries. For
a delicious carob sauce place equal parts unsweetened
carob powder and water in a saucepan and add a dash of
natural peppermint food flavouring. Simmer for about
three minutes, stirring constantly.

Vegetarian cheese
What makes vegetarian cheese different is that the rennet
which is used for curdling the milk has been synthesised by
micro-organisms. Rennet used in non-vegetarian cheese

comes from the contents of the stomach of an unweaned animal, usually a calf. Vegetarian cheese is not suitable for vegans.

Coffee substitutes

In addition to the number of beverages on the market that can be used as substitutes for coffee (see below), dandelion roots may be dried, roasted (until brittle) and ground. All these substitutes are, of course, caffeine-free. Examples of proprietary coffee substitutes include:

1. 'Caro', an instant beverage made from roasted malted barley, barley, chicory and rye.

2. 'Barleycup', made from roasted barley, rye and chicory.

3. 'Prewett's Instant Chicory', made only from soluble extract of roasted chicory root.

Couscous

This is made from durum wheat which has been steamed, cracked and dried. A quick way of making couscous is to pour boiling water over it. Be sure you use enough to adequately cover it with some to spare. In just a few minutes it will be ready to serve with your favourite sauce or seasoning.

Garlic

Most people would not consider garlic to be a fringe food; it is such an important food source, however, that I feel it simply must be included in any book dealing with healthy eating.

Garlic has been known as an important food source and medical aid for thousands of years. According to ancient records it was used at least as early as 3000 BC by a variety of peoples including Babylonians, Chinese, Egyptians, Greeks, Hindus, Romans and Vikings. Culpeper, one of Britain's greatest herbalists, recognised its healing ability.

Paavo Airola, a leading American nutritionist and authority on biological medicine, has spoken to a number of Russian centenarians who all feel that one of the main reasons for their exceptional health and long life is due to the large amounts of garlic and onions in their diets.

Garlic has antibacterial, antifungal and antibiotic properties and the list of ailments that benefit from it is long. It includes: high blood pressure, atherosclerosis, arthritis, diabetes, hypoglycaemia, anaemia, cancer, blood coagulation disorders, sciatica, fungal infections, bronchitis, asthma, allergies, intestinal worms, dysentery, insomnia, troublesome coughs, catarrh, pneumonia, upset stomach, constipation, colds, intestinal disorders. Garlic is also effective in keeping gnats and fleas from getting too friendly!

The most effective way to take garlic is freshly crushed or cut. The problem that some have with the odour can be partly alleviated by mixing it with parsley in salads. Fresh garlic can also be added to sauces, soups and casseroles.

Onions have similar properties to garlic (they belong to the same botanical group) and this makes them another important food source. A warming winter soup can be made from 2 large onions, 2 cloves of garlic, approximately 1½ pints/900 ml of water, 1 oz/25 g miso (see below) and cayenne pepper to taste. Cut each onion in half and slice thinly. Mince the garlic. Boil the water and pour over the miso and stir. Place onions and garlic in a pan and heat until the onions start to soften, constantly stirring to prevent the mixture sticking to the pan (no oil is being used). Pour the miso and water into the pot making sure that all of the miso is removed from the bowl. Add the cayenne to taste, bring to the boil, cover, and allow to simmer for about ½ hour. This makes a delicious and very low-calorie soup.

Herbal teas
There is a wide range of herbal teas to choose from. Some of

the tantalising choices include orange spice, wild strawberry, wild cherry, apple and cinnamon, wild raspberry, lemon grove and almond. Be sure that the label says 'caffeine free'.

Kelp

Kelp is a form of seaweed (dried kombu) which grows among the rocks on most coasts. It is a good source of naturally occurring minerals since it absorbs these from the sea in great abundance. Powdered kelp makes an excellent salt substitute and has the added benefit of aiding weight control (whether loss or gain). It has rather a strong flavour so it is advisable to use less than half the amount of kelp as you would salt.

Kelp is effective for nervous disorders, headaches, high blood pressure, indigestion, and has a stimulating effect on the major organs of the body.

Molasses

Molasses is one of the ingredients removed from sugar cane during the refining process so it contains all the vitamins and minerals that were once part of the total plant. It is best to use brands that are labelled 'unsulphured molasses'. Sulphur is used in the refining process and molasses can contain some of the residue.

Quorn

One of the latest 'alternative foods' to come onto the market, Quorn is advertised as a substitute for meat and is becoming more widely available. A number of pre-packaged meals that contain quorn as an ingredient are also stocked at most major supermarkets.

Quorn is a myco-protein, a distant relative of the mushroom, and has a texture a bit like chicken or prefrozen tofu. Like tofu (below) it is versatile and adopts the flavours of the ingredients it is cooked with. Quorn has only

22 calories per ounce (25 g), has as much protein as an egg of equal weight, contains several of the B vitamins, and is a good source of fibre. In addition, it contains (in descending order of quantity) a number of minerals: phosphorus, potassium, magnesium, calcium, zinc, sodium, copper and iron.

Quorn contains a small quantity of egg white so it is not suitable for vegans.

Royal jelly

This is a milky liquid produced by worker bees in order to nourish the queen bee. The reason why she is greater in size and has a much longer life span than other bees is because she alone is fed exclusively on royal jelly.

Royal jelly contains all the amino acids, which means that it is a complete protein. It contains 10 vitamins (B_1, B_2, B_3, B_5, B_6, B_7, B_8, B_9, B_{12} and C) and six minerals (chromium, iron, manganese, nickel, potassium and sodium). According to Irene Stein in her book *Royal Jelly,* about 4% of the composition of royal jelly remains a mystery, and she feels that it is this unknown factor which causes the failure of any attempt at producing Royal jelly synthetically.

The range of ailments that Ms Stein claims benefits from royal jelly is staggering. Essentially, royal jelly helps the metabolic process and the immune system. It is available in capsules, blended with honey which can be used as a spread, in liquid form, or as a cream for external use.

Seaweed

In addition to kelp (above), other seaweeds available from any good health shop include:

Arame – this usually comes in black spaghetti-like strips and has a shrimp-like flavour. It contains calcium and phosphorus.

Dulse – a red seaweed with a tangy flavour when dried. It

can also be soaked and used as an addition to savoury dishes. Contains potassium and magnesium as well as other minerals.

Hijiki – will expand quite a bit when soaked in hot water (takes about 15 minutes). Contains vitamins A, B_1, B_2, calcium, selenium, magnesium, iron and zinc.

Nori – comes in flat paper-thin sheets which are good lightly toasted, giving it a crisp texture and nutty flavour. A good source of protein and also contains vitamins A, B_2, B_{12}, D and niacin.

Wakame – available dried, it is best soaked in hot water to soften it before using. High in calcium.

Seaweed can be used in soups, salads, stir-fried dishes and casseroles. Nori makes a good snack when eaten dried.

Soya products

The soya bean is the only legume which is a complete protein (it contains all the essential amino acids). Soya beans also contain vitamin A, many B vitamins, vitamins C, D and E, fibre, potassium, phosphorus, iron and calcium. Soya beans are one of the few vegetable sources of Omega-3 fatty acids and lecithin. Miso and tempeh, made from soya, contain B_{12} as a result of the fermentation process. The versatility of the soya bean is unique and some of the products made from it are as follows:

Miso – made from fermented soya beans and sea salt. Miso is a savoury seasoning that has a texture resembling soft peanut butter. The length of fermentation time will determine the colour and flavour. Uses include: bouillon for soups, stock for vegetarian stew, seasoning similar to Worcestershire sauce.

Okara – a blend of puréed, soaked soya beans left over from the production of soya milk and tofu. Okara is rich in fibre as well as protein and can be used in burgers, pâtés, cakes, etc.

Shoyu sauce – made from fermented soya beans and wheat which gives it a slightly milder flavour than tamari.

Soya dessert – a low calorie dessert option which contains dehulled soya beans, raw cane sugar, maize starch, sea-weed, sea salt and natural flavourings (vanilla, strawberry, chocolate, banana and carob). (*Note:* the carob used here does not contain sugar, which means it contains fewer calories than the other choices.)

Soya flakes – produced by running lightly dry-roasted whole soya beans through a roller mill; this makes the soya beans easier to use in cooking.

Soya flour – a finely textured flour, pale yellow in colour, which is a key ingredient for protein-rich breads. However, because soya flour does not contain gluten it is necessary to mix it with other flours to obtain the desired texture when making breads, cakes, etc.

Soya milk – based on protein from the soya bean and therefore allowable for milk-free diets. The manufacturers Unisoy make a product called 'Gold Soya Milk' which is made from organic soya beans and sweetened only with apple juice. They also produce 'Ice Supreme' (ice cream substitute) made from organic soya milk and sweetened with apple juice.

Soya oil – the oil from the bean is rich in polyunsaturates.

Soya sauce/Tamari – a light or dark brown liquid which is made from fermented soya beans and sea salt and may contain caramel colouring. Tamari is a pure soy sauce.

Tofu – also known as bean curd, tofu has been used in parts of Asia for over 2000 years; it is still, however, considered an 'alternative' or 'new fangled' food in the West! Tofu is made by curdling the 'milk' of the soya bean to separate out the solids. Tofu is an excellent food source, especially for vegans and vegetarians, because it is high in protein, low in calories and fats and contains no cholesterol. Tofu looks like either solid cottage cheese (the firm variety) or custard (the silken variety) and comes packaged in water. The very mild, almost non-existent taste of tofu makes it one of the most versatile food sources available. The skill in cooking with tofu has to do with the ingredients used with it. It can be used equally as the base for dips and desserts (silken variety), or for savoury dishes like tofu burgers, lasagne, chilli con carne, and so on (firm variety). Tofu is a food source truly worth experimenting with. (See Bibliography for some excellent tofu cookbooks.)

Tempeh – fermented tofu which contains vitamin B_{12}, which is lacking in some vegetarian and vegan diets. Its unique flavour makes it a welcome addition to salads (used as a crouton substitute), or added to pizza, stir-fried rice dishes or casseroles.

Textured vegetable protein (TVP) – an excellent meat substitute because of its chewy nature. TVP can be purchased in nugget- or mince-sized pieces. It needs to be reconstituted (by soaking in water) prior to use. TVP is available in healthfood shops and supermarkets but can also be made at home from pre-frozen tofu and tamari. The tofu, once thawed, needs to be cut into small cubes or chopped (depending on the texture desired) and placed in a bowl with the tamari poured over it. Use about four tablespoons tamari to 1 lb/450 g tofu. Mix to ensure that the tamari has been fully absorbed, spread on a baking sheet, and bake for about one hour or until the tofu is completely dry (300°F, 150°C, gas mark 2). After cooling, the TVP can be stored in an airtight container until you are ready to use it. To use, all you have to do is pour boiling water over the desired amount and let stand for about 15 minutes.

Bean sprouts

When seeds of plants such as beans are soaked in water enzymes are activated which enhance the nutrient value of the seed. In effect, these 'sprouted' seeds are predigested and the body's own enzymes are stimulated by such foods. Sprouts are higher in nutrients weight for weight than any other food source.

Sprouting can easily be done at home. Use a bowl with one or more holes at the base or a strainer placed over a bowl. Place the beans (or whatever you are going to use) in the bowl or strainer and at least once a day pour water over them. Once the water has soaked through into the larger bowl it can be removed. Within two to three days the sprouts should be ready to eat; they make a wonderful addition to salads or a crisp sandwich.

Dried beans and pulses (such as mung, lentils, aduki, chickpeas, etc.), seeds (such as sunflower, sesame, pumpkin), and alfalfa are all ideal for sprouting.

Tahini

This is a creamy paste made from ground sesame seeds and sesame oil. Sesame seeds are high in calcium and protein. They also contain phosphorus in about the proportion to calcium that the body requires. Tahini makes a wonderful spread on crackers or used in recipes as a peanut butter replacement.

Wheatgerm

The richest source of vitamin E is found in wheatgerm. It also contains vitamin B-complex. It can be sprinkled on cereals, salads, casseroles, desserts, etc.

Yoghurt

The fermenting process of the milk enhances its nutritional value by allowing the proteins, milk sugars and calcium to become more readily available. A number of the health benefits provided by bacteria – such as vitamin synthesis as well as anticarcinogenic, antiviral, antifungal and detoxification qualities – are available when live cultures are used. The cultures *L. bulgaricus* and *S. thermophilus* are needed to produce 'real' yoghurt according to Leon Chaitow, a leader in the field of alternative health. He warns (in *Here's Health*, March, 1990) that most yoghurts sold do not contain any of these qualities, and, since there is no legislation which stipulates what cultures must be used as starter organisms, if you want the real thing it is important to find out what you are actually buying. *It is important to read the label to ensure that the yoghurt is live and the proper cultures are used.*

Other products available
There are an increasing number of products available that are organic and/or contain only natural ingredients. Sometimes just 'an impression' of naturalness is given, so even if a product is bought in a health store, it is still important to read the label with extreme care.

Although it is impossible to provide a list of all the products currently available that are made from high quality ingredients, I have included a list of some of the products available at the time of writing:

The New Covent Garden Soup Company – produce an excellent range of soups including 'Mushroom with Garlic', 'Spinach with Nutmeg' and 'Carrot and Coriander'.

Various producers of decaffeinated teas – a number of these are now available and obtainable from most supermarkets.

Unisoy – in addition to their regular soya milk products, this company produces a carob and banana organic drink which satisfies the sweet tooth (it is sweetened with organic raw cane molasses).

Martlet – producers of organic cider vinegar and other products.

Meridian – make a peanut butter that contains no added sugar or palm oil. It is made from roasted peanuts and sea salt (less than 1%).

Life – produce a number of all-natural products including tomato ketchup with cider vinegar and Worcestershire sauce. Their products contain no added sugar or salt.

Goodness Foods – produce a variety of packaged organic wholefoods which includes a range of dried fruits, seeds, nuts and pulses, popcorn, brown rice, muesli.

Granose – in addition to many other products, Granose now produce an organic baby food which comes in eight varieties, of which four are free from gluten. They are all suitable for vegetarians.

Tivall – produce a number of meat substitute vegetarian products including burger, schnitzel, sausage, sausage roll and savoury strüdel.

If any of the above products are not available from your grocery, ask for them at your healthfood shop. If they do not stock them, ask them why not.

▶ GO TO ▶ ◆ *Food ecology, page 217*

17 Food safety

The concerns over food safety that have been voiced in the alternative health field for many years have finally started to get through to the majority. This has occurred not only as a result of the hard work and research carried on over the years by many dedicated and knowledgeable people in this field, but to a considerable extent because of a statement made by the then Junior Minister of Health proclaiming that most eggs carried salmonella. This comment was pounced on by the press, setting wheels in motion that brought the whole issue of food safety to the fore. As a result, other problem areas were also brought to light, although Edwina Currie, the Junior Minister responsible for the statement, lost her job.

The furore that erupted over the weeks following the salmonella issue, which also brought up concerns about listeria and BSE (bovine spongiform encephalopathy), has abated, but public concern over food safety has nevertheless been alerted.

There are a number of factors that can cause food spoilage. Most common are bacteria, moulds and yeasts, all of which grow rapidly at temperatures around 10°C to 60°C (50°F to 140°F) where moisture is available. In many cases, this growth can be retarded by refrigeration and arrested by freezing.

There are about 2000 strains of salmonella, of which about 1200 are capable of causing illness in humans. Salmonella enteritidis is usually associated with poultry. Surveys have shown that six or seven out of every 10 oven-ready chickens contain salmonella.

It is almost impossible to know how many eggs are contaminated with salmonella at any given time. Until poultry farmers become convinced of the importance of hygienic practice (see Chapter 18), we can best protect ourselves by ensuring that all the poultry, eggs and meat we consume is adequately cooked and not allowed to stand around too long at room temperature before it is either eaten or refrigerated. It is also important to keep raw foods such as uncooked chicken or eggs from getting into contact with other food items. Utensils used when working with these raw foods should be thoroughly cleaned before being re-used.

Although listeria, another micro-organism, is not as common as salmonella, the increase in the use of cook-chilled meals (unless they are used properly) may change that. These foods are pre-cooked and then chilled to a temperature which must be between 0 and 3 degrees centigrade. The cook-chilled meal must be adequately reheated prior to eating to ensure that any potential pathogenic bacteria is destroyed. Other foods that can carry listeria include soft cheese and shellfish. Vegetables may also be a carrier and they should always be washed prior to usage, especially if they are to be eaten raw. For the most part, however, a healthy body should be resistant to listeria.

These are just a few examples of what can happen to food if care is not taken in handling and preparation. *BBC Food Check*, by David Edwards (Food Hygiene Bureau) and Peter Bazalgette, is, as the subtitle suggests, a 'practical guide to safe food' and well worth reading as it goes into the kind of detail that there is no space for here.

An important factor to remember is that while we have control over what goes on in our own kitchen, eating out is quite a different matter. There are no guarantees (although there are legal safeguards as a result of the new Food Safety Act) that the people handling the food we order will take, or are even aware of, the proper care required.

ADDITIVES AND PRESERVATIVES

The additives and preservatives that manufacturers put into packaged foods serve a number of purposes. The main one, obviously, is to retard, or in some cases prevent, food spoilage thus ensuring that the food is preserved and has a prolonged shelf life. Some preservatives, as well as colourings, have been shown to cause dramatic emotional changes in consumers of foods containing them.

Additives may be used to aid in the processing or preparation of the food or simply to enhance its flavour or appearance. In some cases additives are used to improve nutritional value, usually because nutrients occurring naturally have been removed as a result of the processing procedure.

Since 1986, most packaged food displays a list of the ingredients contained in the product. However, unless you happen to be a chemist, the contents can still remain a mystery. And then there are the E numbers (codes for food additives which have been approved by the European Community and are standard for all food manufacturers in the EC — see Table 8).

Table 8: Additive and preservative E-number groupings

E100–E180	Food colourings
E200–E297	Preservatives
E300–E320	Antioxidants
E321–545	Emulsifiers, stabilisers, etc.*
551–576	Anti-caking agents*
577–900	Flavour enhancers*
901–907	Glazing agents*
920–927	Improving agents*

* some of these numbers are not yet classified as E numbers but are under consideration by the EC.

The importance of understanding what added extras are included in the products that we eat, and what implications they can have, cannot be overstressed. For example, starches are used as thickeners. 'Modified starch' is a term that means the starch has been chemically changed. At present modified starches do not need E numbers. As consumers we are entitled to know exactly what it is that we are putting into our bodies. Manufacturers ought voluntarily to inform us by comprehensive labelling on food items — labels which include *all* the ingredients. It is worth bearing in mind that we do have the choice of not purchasing items if they are not properly labelled. It is our right to know what ingredients a food contains and what they do or don't do to us.

FOOD COLOURINGS

There are a number of reasons why manufacturers feel that they have to artificially colour certain foods. In the case of canned foods, the heat used in the process causes much of the natural colour of the food to be lost. Rather than have a consumer turn away from a product because it appears to be artificial in colour, the food is artificially coloured 'to make it look like it is supposed to'.

Fish flesh too can be coloured. The normal life cycle of a salmon starts in fresh water prior to journeying down river, often over incredible distances, to a salt water environment. After a number of years the salmon is somehow drawn back to its birthplace in order to spawn. The natural pink colour of salmon comes from a particular type of shrimp which forms part of its diet. However, most of the salmon that reach our plates are factory farmed and obtain their pink colour from artificial colourants. To ensure that the pink is an acceptable colour, they are sometimes starved for several weeks before they are 'harvested'.

In other instances, colour may simply be added to a food

that would otherwise be colourless, as in the case of instant desserts or ice lollies, to make them attractive to the consumer.

There are 16 artificial colours that are acceptable for use in the UK, compared to seven in the United States. In Norway, the use of artificial colour is non-existent. Although these colours are considered to be safe, there has been a lot of controversy with certain ones, particularly E110 (sunset yellow) and E102 (tartrazine). Both of these colourings are derived from synthetic azo dyes, which causes sensitivity in a proportion of the population, usually in the form of contractions of the bronchial tubes. It is believed by some researchers that the artificial orange colour used in such items as fizzy drinks plays a major role in causing hyperactivity, usually in children.

The question is really why is it necessary to add colour at all? An informed consumer who does not expect food to be highly coloured is surely a better alternative.

PRESERVATIVES

There are a number of ways to protect foods from spoiling. Although canned foods enjoy a long shelf-life, many of the vitamins, minerals and enzymes are lost as a result of the heat process that is required for sterilisation in the first place. When water is removed from foods (dried fruits, for example) a vitamin loss will also occur. Although nutrients generally remain intact as a result of freezing, the texture of the food can be altered.

There is a lot of controversy when it comes to cook-chilled foods (see above). It is recommended that the food be reheated within five days and eaten at one sitting (no leftovers). There is a risk of contamination if careful manufacturing procedures are not followed.

Preservatives are often added to foods in order to prolong shelf life by retarding the growth of bacteria, fungi and viruses. In some cases preservatives are used to protect the natural colour or flavour of the food. Alas, however, most of the preservatives used are synthetically produced and can cause problems for people not in optimal health. Out of the 46 preservatives described in Maurice Hanssen's book, *E For Additives*, 15 contain warnings for people with asthma or related breathing problems, 11 have skin sensitivity warnings and the Hyperactive Children's Support Group recommends that 18 of them be avoided. There are other warnings associated with many of the preservatives listed, making it well worthwhile to have a copy of Hanssen's book to hand.

Sulphur dioxide is one of the oldest food additives known and was used by the Egyptians as a preservative for wine. Although it occurs naturally it can also be produced synthetically. Today it is used as a bleaching agent for flour, in dough for the manufacturing of biscuits, and in the malting process for beer. Sulphur dioxide was widely used in the USA to spray the vegetables in salad bars in order to keep them looking fresh. A number of deaths from asthma in the United States were linked with its excessive use. The importance of being aware of preservative use is obvious. What may not be so obvious is the number of different food items that actually contain them. Although label reading can add quite a bit to the time necessary for food shopping, it is indeed time well spent.

ANTIOXIDANTS

When certain foods are exposed to oxygen, chemical changes in the food can occur. This is easily demonstrated by leaving a freshly cut apple on a plate for a few minutes. The fruit will start to turn a light brown colour as a result of oxidation. The placing of lemon juice on a freshly cut apple will retard the oxidation process. The vitamin C (ascorbic acid) present in the lemon acts as an antioxidant and this stops the apple discolouring.

Fats and oils can become rancid if they are exposed to oxygen for a lengthy period of time. Digestion of foods containing rancid fats or oils can cause illness. Using antioxidants in oils and fats can prevent or delay the oxidation process.

Vitamin E, another naturally occurring antioxidant, is removed from vegetable oils, unless they are cold-pressed, during the refining process.

A number of different antioxidants are used to prevent oxidation; a few of these (like vitamin E, above) are natural, but many more are synthetic and can have side effects.

EMULSIFIERS AND STABILISERS

Emulsifiers are used to combine substances that do not, under normal circumstances, mix, such as oil and water, to create a smooth consistency in a product. Lecithin (E322) most commonly obtained from soya beans, is a good example of a natural emulsifier.

Stabilisers ensure that the substances that have been combined, usually by emulsifiers, do not separate. They help to improve the texture of the product.

Other related additives that fall under this category include:

• buffers – chemical substances which can control the acid/alkali balance;
• firming agents – prevent food from breaking up during processing;
• raising agents – allow aeration to occur which can increase volume and decrease density;
• sequestrants – substances which prevent trace metals from causing foods to oxidise;
• synergists – substances which can enhance the effect of other substances such as antioxidants.

ANTI-CAKING AGENTS

These additives prevent lumps occurring in powdered and crystalline substances (such as icing sugar and salt) by controlling moisture.

FLAVOURS AND FLAVOUR ENHANCERS

These are used in foods to restore flavours lost in processing, or simply to exaggerate the flavours that already exist. The source of 'flavours' can be extracts or essential oils, whereas 'flavour enhancers' are usually always from a synthetic source. Probably the most well-known flavour enhancer is monosodium glutamate (MSG), which is the sodium salt of glutamic acid, a naturally occurring amino acid. However, MSG is usually manufactured by fermentation using molasses from cane or beet sugar. It is used to increase the flavour of proteins.

One of the most deceptive aspects of labelling is the use of the word 'flavour'. For example, if the word 'banana' simply appears by itself on a label's ingredient list, then the product is made with real bananas; if the term 'banana flavoured' is used, however, that means that although a significant part of the flavour must be from bananas, it need not be totally from that source. The most important thing to remember, however, is that if the words 'banana *flavour*' appear on the packet, then the product will probably not contain any real bananas at all!

According to the *Look at the Label* booklet which is produced by the Ministry of Agriculture, Fisheries and Food, 'Labels must state that flavourings have been used but need not list them by name'. If manufacturers choose to simply use the word 'flavourings' rather than indicating exactly what is in the product, this only begs the question — why?

With the wide variety of herbs and spices available it is

difficult to understand why artificial flavour enhancers are necessary. As for flavours — well, if it is the taste of strawberry that you want, why not use the real thing?

GLAZING AGENTS

These substances provide a shine or 'protective' coating on the surface of foods. Some glazing agents can cause skin irritation.

IMPROVING AGENTS

These are used mainly in flour and can help to create a lighter and softer product, as in bread. Chlorine (925) or chlorine dioxide (synthetically prepared; 926) may be used as a bleaching agent and as an antibacterial and antifungal preservative in flour. Unfortunately, much of the naturally occurring vitamin E is destroyed in the process.

Shortly prior to writing this, it was announced that MAFF was to ban potassium bromate (924) because, based on rat experiments, it proved to be a cancer risk. This substance is used mainly in white bread to give it a lighter, softer quality. The report went on to say that there have been doubts about this particular additive since 1974!

SWEETENERS

Sweeteners, as the name implies, are added to foods to give them a sweet flavour. Sugar is the most commonly known sweetener. The Oxford dictionary definition of sugar is – 'kinds of sweet crystalline substance prepared from cane, beet and other plants for use in cookery, confectionery ...'. Unfortunately, during refining, all of the fibre, protein and other nutrients naturally occurring in the plants are removed, leaving nothing of nutritional value. Sugar can best be classified as an additive because the only thing it has to offer is quick energy from the calories it contains. In order for sugar to be digested, vitamins and minerals must be taken from cells in the body. The more sugar that is consumed, the less essential nutrients are available for carrying out other vital functions. The over-consumption of sugar is felt by many to be the underlying cause in a number of diseases including diabetes and hypoglycaemia (see Chapter 4).

Sucrose is a carbohydrate consisting of glucose and fructose. It is the principle constituent of cane sugar and sugar beet and is what is commonly known as sugar. Brown sugar is made from white refined sugar with some molasses (see Chapter 16) re-added to obtain the brown colour.

Other sweeteners include:

• corn syrup – derived from cornstarch; contains no nutritional value;
• maple syrup – 65% sucrose and contains some nutrients;
• honey – probably the first sweetener ever used. Having been predigested by the bees, it is already a simple sugar. It is many times sweeter than sugar, hence less is needed. Unlike sugar, about one quarter of the contents of honey consists of minerals, vitamins and important trace substances. The darker the honey, the more of these nutrients are present. Through processing, however, some of the nutritional value is lost. Although honey contains dextrose, which is absorbed into the blood quickly, other sugar properties are more slowly absorbed, allowing a steady level of blood sugar concentration to be maintained. If, however, the honey is heat-processed at a temperature of above 117°F, the sugars start to break down and can end up as no more beneficial than refined white sugar. It is best to obtain raw honey, which is usually sold by local farms or in healthfood shops;
• aspartame – an artificial sweetener of protein origin

usually found in confectionery, ice cream, low-calorie desserts and soft drinks;

• fructose – naturally occurring in fruit and honey;

• glucose (dextrose) – an additive derived from cornstarch. It is less expensive than sugar, contains about the same amount of calories, but is not as sweet; larger amounts may therefore be used;

• maltose – made from grain starch; the molecules are broken down into sugar as a result of the malting process. Barley malt and rice syrup are two examples;

• lactose – the sugar found naturally in milk and milk products;

• invert sugar – a sugar made from 50% glucose and 50% fructose;

• saccharin – discovered in 1879. Derived from coal-tar and approximately 400 times sweeter than sugar. Although it is calorie free, it has a bitter aftertaste. Because it is destroyed by heat it is not used in cooking. Often used as a sweetener for diabetic and low-calorie foods.

In the 1950s another coal-tar derivative became popular in the United States. The panacea for the sweet tooth, a calorie free sweetener without a bitter aftertaste and heat-resistant so it could be used in cooking — enter cyclamates. Widespread use of cyclamates took their toll in a number of ways. Among the adverse reactions were damage to fetuses, inhibited growth, kidney, liver and intestinal problems, and changes in blood coagulation, to name but a few. In October 1969, 19 years after their introduction, cyclamates were banned in the USA.

FOOD LABELLING

In a perfect society we would be able to go into any food store and pick up any item from the shelf feeling confident that it was of the finest quality, containing only pure ingredients. What else would a shopkeeper have on the shelf? Certainly all shops are concerned about the quality of the items they sell, aren't they? Alas, as we know only too well, we do not live in a perfect society. It is up to each of us to ensure that what we purchase is in fact good for us.

It is important, of course, to know how to read the labels when they are available, as sometimes the information can be a bit misleading. Firstly, all of the ingredients listed must be in descending order by weight. The problem is, how can we be sure that ALL of the ingredients are listed? For example, many ingredients lists will simply say 'herbs' or 'spices' without listing specifically *which* herbs or spices. It is just as important to know that nutmeg is an ingredient in a product as it is to know that milk is, particularly if you happen to be allergic to it! If there is water in the product, it need only be included on the ingredients list if it accounts for more than 5% of the total weight.

A very important point to remember is that just because a product says it is strawberry something-or-other does not mean that anything resembling a real strawberry is part of the product, unless, of course, 'strawberry' is listed on the ingredients list (see above). There is usually no telling which of the unpronounceable words that may be listed are the ingredients that add the strawberry-like flavour to the product.

When a product says 'sugar free' or 'no added sugar' it is still a good idea to give a quick check to the ingredients list to determine if the product is sweetened at all, and if so by what. Sugar is most commonly equated with sucrose. However, there are a number of forms that sugar takes and so it is important to know that such ingredients as corn syrup, fructose, dextrose and glucose, if present in the ingredients list, mean that the product is not really without any form of sugar.

It should go without saying that it is important to check the use-by date or the best-before date on the package before purchase. Substantial price reductions are often made on products that have reached or slightly gone over their sell-by date. There is no reason not to take advantage of the lower prices, providing that the product is used fairly soon after purchase.

Some labels will include nutritional information, although that rarely includes information regarding the vitamin and mineral content of a product. The information provided is often based on a particular weight, say a serving size. In some cases the information relates to the entire contents of the package. It is important to understand what the amounts relate to, especially if you are calorie counting. It is easy to assume that the information provided is for the entire package, whereas it is usually for only a portion of it. The information normally includes:

Calories – usually labelled as 'energy'. The actual calorie number is usually given in 'kcal' (kilocalories) per 100 g;

Protein – usually given in g/100 g;

Carbohydrate – usually given in g/100 g. The total amount (which consists of starches and sugars) is sometimes followed by the amount which consists of sugar;

Fat – usually given in g/100 g. The total amount of fat is sometimes followed by the amount which consists of saturated fat;

Fibre – usually given in g/100 g;

Sodium (salt) – usually given in g (or parts of a gram)/ 100 g.

The total amount of food, excluding the packaging, is required to be shown in metric units, grams. This total amount may not be the same as the weight used on the nutritional information panel, as indicated above.

Specific storage and usage instructions may be provided: what temperature is necessary for heating the product; the length of time required for cooking (time indicated for microwaves can vary based on the wattage of the machine); preparation instructions if other ingredients are required.

Although there are certain laws which govern the amount of meat which must be present in a meat pie, other factors such as the percentage of lean meat and the indication of what part(s) of the carcass make up the remaining percentage, are not mandatory. The nature of the contents can then be disguised by the use of flavour enhancers for taste and red food colouring which allows the meat to appear leaner than might actually be the case.

Chocolate is another interesting case. Although ingredients are listed on the outside wrapper of a large package (of six Mars bars, for instance), the individually-wrapped bars lack this information. This means that when bars are purchased separately the complete ingredients list is nowhere to be found. This is true of almost every individual chocolate bar. The Swiss chocolate manufacturer, Toblerone, does have an ingredients list, in a number of languages, on each individual package. Yet even here, because the name 'Toblerone' is superimposed in large letters directly over this information, it makes it difficult to read.

In bygone days when a food (usually meat) was smoked it meant that it was hung in a chimney, usually after being salted. This added flavour to the meat and also helped to preserve it by inhibiting bacterial growth. Today the term 'smoked' may simply mean that the meat or fish has been dipped in liquid smoke flavour and probably artificially coloured. If the food is pre-packaged it should clearly be stated, but in the case of unpackaged food this may not be so obvious.

Foods such as those purchased from a bakery rarely have ingredient information because they do not come pre-wrapped. That really should not be a determining factor and somehow the information should be available, at least upon request. Just because the product may be made on the premises does not necessarily mean that the ingredients used are beyond doubt.

There is also the whole question of residues from pesticides and fungicides that may be present, especially where vegetables, fruits and grains make up all or part of the product.

By law, there are restrictions on claims that manufacturers can make for their products. For example, claims may only be made for vitamins and minerals if those vitamins and minerals are listed in one of two schedules provided for under the Food Labelling Regulations and they meet certain percentages of the minimum daily requirements set out by the regulations.

FOOD IRRADIATION

The most frightening and controversial aspect of 'food safety', now legal, is food irradiation. The concept is that rather than using chemical additives, food can be preserved by using doses of ionising radiation. This causes chemical changes to the food, such as the destruction of the enzymes that ripen fruit, and inhibits the sprouting of some root vegetables. Shelf life is thus prolonged and this reduces waste. In addition, certain bacteria which might otherwise cause food poisoning are killed by the process. On the surface this looks like an ideal answer to food preservation. Or is it just an ideal mechanism for additional profits?

There are a number of questions about food irradiation that have yet to be satisfactorily answered. One of the most important is how can the consumer be assured that because the food being purchased has been irradiated it is not just covering up the fact that unhygienic processing has occurred or poor quality food has been used which would otherwise be unsaleable? Foods that have been untampered with have built in warning systems, an example being potatoes turning green. Irradiation masks these warning systems. Also, there has been little consideration given to the effects that irradiation has on foods that have already been treated with pesticides and other chemicals such as additives.

Irradiation also reduces the nutritional value of the food. Specific vitamins at risk are vitamins A, B_1 (thiamine), B_2 (riboflavin), B_3 (niacin), B_6, B_{12}, C, E, K, and folic acid. Losses can vary from 20% to 80% in some foods. These losses, of course, occur over and above any losses due to cooking and storage of the foods involved, and in some cases the irradiation of the food actually increases the amount of loss during storage. Since one of the benefits of irradiation is supposed to be increased storage time, vitamin losses in certain foods can be quite significant.

The main foods being targetted for irradiation are fresh fruits, vegetables and whole grains. Because fats tend to develop a rancid flavour and odour when irradiated, items such as red meat, milk and milk products will probably not become candidates for the process.

Since it is impossible to tell whether or not food has been irradiated it is hoped that adequate labelling will be provided to allow consumers the option of purchasing or not purchasing these products. However, from a strictly pragmatic point of view, surely not enough long-term testing has been even considered, let alone conducted, to make it feasible for food irraditation to be put into practice? What effect on the body do the free radicals resulting from the chemical changes brought about by the irradiation process have?

The main question asked by Tony Webb and Tim Lang of The London Food Commission in their excellent book, *Food Irradiation*, is: 'If any food had to be irradiated, what was wrong with it?' A good question. A sharper one was made by Richard Piccioni in *The Ecologist* (Vol. 18, No. 2, 1988) when he asks whether the irradiation of food is 'an unscrupulous attempt to find a commercial use for nuclear wastes'?

▶ GO TO ▶   ◆ *Food ecology, page 217.*

18 *Food ecology*

Two major problems plague our world and should be the prime concern and responsibility of each one of us. These fundamental problems are: (a) people all over the world are dying from starvation or at least suffering malnutrition, and (b) pollution affects the water that we use, the air that we breathe and the planet that we inhabit. Although these problems may seem overwhelming, there actually are things that each one of us can do, if we choose to, to help change both these situations.

It may seem hard to believe but each time we go food shopping we influence both these problems. Depending on the choices that we make, we are actually alleviating or helping to perpetuate them by a tiny amount. Compound that by the hundreds of millions of consumers in the First World, and we are talking about a big effect.

It is now common knowledge that eating too much fat is directly linked to heart disease, the most common cause of death in the UK. Government committees to bodies such as the British Medical Association recommend a significant reduction in the amount of saturated fats in the average British diet. The main food culprits are meat and dairy products because of the high amount of saturated fat that they contain. Further information on the connection between meat and animal by-products and the potential for heart disease should be readily available from your local practitioner whether alternative or orthodox. The British Nutrition Foundation also produces a helpful booklet, *Eating for a Healthier Heart* (see Useful addresses). But there are some lesser-known facts about meat and animal by-products that many people feel are of equal importance when making choices at the grocers. One of these is the factory farming methods that directly account for the abundance of meat available.

Because we sometimes see animals such as cows and sheep quietly grazing in the fields, we are somehow lulled into assuming that all farm animals enjoy such a lifestyle. In fact, the creatures that provide most of the meat that ends up on the dinner table – the majority of farm animals – have an existence as far removed from such a pastoral idyll as Mickey Mouse is from becoming President of the United States. Many of the chickens, pigs and calves destined for human consumption never see the light of day.

Piglets are snatched from their mothers when they are about three weeks old and sometimes placed in wire mesh cages for several weeks. They end up being crammed together for the 'fattening up' process. To avoid too much damage from biting one another's tails due to the frustration of their condition, their teeth are pulled and tails routinely docked. When the piglet is of the required weight, 24 weeks or more after birth, it is ready to be sent for slaughter. In the meantime, the sows are probably already pregnant with the next batch because that process starts immediately upon separation from their piglets. For a full detailed account of the sacrifice made by the pigs that provide most of the bacon, ham or pork meals, a four-page report entitled *Pig's Diary* is available from Animal Aid (see Useful addresses).

Broiler chickens (the kind we eat) spend their seven or so weeks of life packed into sheds by the thousands. There they are fattened, sometimes to the point that they have difficulty walking, prior to being slaughtered.

To obtain the 'special-fed' status that gourmets look for in veal, calves are separated from their mothers several days after birth and spend the rest of their approximately 16-week life, sometimes chained by the neck, in a crate not big enough for them to turn around in. These animals are kept separated from each other and in darkness with nothing but the floor to either lie on or stand up on. In order to give the veal that 'milk-fed' look, the calves are fed a diet that is deficient in iron, making them anaemic.

Animals are often given doses of antibiotics to prevent infectious diseases from occurring as a result of the appalling conditions they are forced to endure. Continually eating meat laced with antibiotics can cause a reduction in the effectiveness of the very antibiotics that may one day be prescribed for a serious illness.

One of the latest 'scientific advances' is the preparation bovine somatotrophin (BST), a genetically-engineered growth hormone. BST boosts milk yield by an average of 10–25%. It is claimed by the pharmaceutical industry that milk quality is not affected and that there are no traces of the increased hormone levels in the final product. Use of the drug involves injecting the cows once every two weeks. According to an article in the *Ecologist* (Sept/Oct, 1989), secret field tests are being carried out at ten farms in different parts of Britain. There is a lot of controversy surrounding the use of this drug. The *Ecologist* report explores a wide range of opinion on the subject, including an article from the *Journal of Dairy Science*, 1984, by J. Bitman *et al*, which claims that hormones can induce a wide range of measurable changes in milk composition. It says that up to 27% higher fat levels have been noted in BST-treated milk. This seems to contradict the pharmaceutical industry's claims. As of this writing BST has not yet been approved for use.

In addition to providing calves for meat, dairy cows provide the milk their calves are deprived of. They are actually forced to produce more milk than would normally be required by their offspring by being fed high protein concentrates to increase milk yield. The fact that ingesting too much of these concentrates can lead to lameness does not seem to be a cause of concern. Neither does the mastitis (painful inflammation of the udder), suffered by approximately one third of the dairy cows. Mastitis is caused by machine milking and indoor cubicle housing.

BSE (bovine spongiform encephalopathy) is another fairly recent problem that has manifested in the beef herd. Basically it seems to be a disease of the brain which has been affecting cows all over the country. The disease was first recognised in 1986 and by February 1989 there were more than 2500 known cases. Although there is no evidence that the disease is transmissible from cows to humans there is no common consensus on the ultimate risk factor. The problem seems to stem from the early 1980s when cattle feed started to be supplemented with offals from the abattoir. It is believed that the brains from sheep which were infected by scrapie, a sheep brain disease similar to BSE, were used. The problem was exacerbated when offals were processed at lower temperatures which failed to kill off the virus. A ban has been levied on this procedure. (Many people were shocked to learn that herbivores like cattle were being fed animal protein at all.)

The use of organic feed for animals is as important for them as it is for us — and for us in any case if we eat them in turn! Organically raised chickens will not be fed the salmonella-infected remains of battery hens, for example. Another thing to keep in mind is that most organ meat will be infected with toxins unless the animals are also fed organically. This is particularly true for liver, since the liver in an animal performs the same process as it does in a human: the liver deals with toxins by filtering them out of the blood and storing them in its tissue. The liver can therefore be loaded with toxins just waiting to be processed for human consumption. Toxic residues provide yet another reason for eating only lean meat: just like us, toxins in animals can also be stored in the fat.

Battery hens are another victim of factory farming methods. They are crowded, often five to a cage, into a space which is only 18 in/45 cm by 20 in/50 cm. These cages are often stacked one on top of another. There is no room for the hens to spread their wings. They are denied the right to express normal hen behaviour patterns such as dust-bathing, ground scratching and nesting. Instead they are forced to stand all day and night on a sloping wire mesh floor. They must strain their necks to reach the feed that comes to them on conveyor belts. The top third of the beak is often cut off for their protection. This is so that the hens do not hurt one another out of frustration due to the appalling conditions they are subjected to. The life span of a battery hen is usually about a year. At this point her egg-laying capability has tailed off and she is sent to be slaughtered.

Large scale factory farming exists because of the demand for meat and dairy products at a low price. But what is the source of the demand? We are taught that there are four basic food groups: meat; dairy; grains; fruit and vegetables. Because of this many people naturally assume that half of their daily diet should be made up of meat and dairy products. Considering that a good proportion of the nutritional information given out in, say, schools, comes from the dairy and meat industries, there is a rather obvious question that needs answering — is this information biased? A positive answer to this question necessitates further inquiry. For example, perhaps part of standard education should be mandatory visits to at least one factory farm and abbatoir.

There are other reasons why factory farming methods need to be re-evaluated. Rearing animals for food is not an efficient method of food supply. Producing crops on agricultural land currently used for the raising of animals strictly for meat supply could go a long way towards helping to eliminate hunger, particularly in Third World countries. Staggering statistics suggest that animals are fed over 80% of the total grain crops grown in Western countries. In *Diet for a New America*, John Robbins claims that for 'every sixteen pounds of grain and soya beans fed to beef cattle, we get back only one pound as meat on our plates'. So why do we choose to let people starve when the solution could be so simple?

Further, traditional crops that were once raised in Third World countries, and which were often ideally suited to the local conditions, have been abandoned in favour of crops like coffee and cocoa which are suitable for export, particularly because of Western demand — and Third World debt to First World banks.

WHY ORGANIC?

There are guidelines that can tell us what vitamins and minerals can be found in particular foods. However, it is impossible for us to know exactly how much of a particular vitamin or mineral we get from a particular piece of fruit, vegetable, meat, etc. It is a fact that food which has been grown on soils treated with a variety of chemical sprays will be robbed of many of the nutrients that they might have otherwise contained. Likewise, animals which are fed on crops grown in nutrient-deficient soils will not produce the same quality of meat as organically fed livestock. For fruit and vegetables, consideration must also be given to the time lapse between picking and eating. If not eaten raw, cooking methods must also be considered. All of these things add to the decreased nutritional value of the foods that we eat.

Fruits and vegetables, organic or not, that are exposed to exhaust from vehicles may be contaminated with lead. This can be as a result of street display stands or fields that are too close to roads or railways.

Current agricultural practices seem to be at the root of a number of increasingly dangerous situations: levels of nitrates, for example, in food and water are rising. Nitrates are essential to plant growth, and adding more to the soil can increase overall productivity. They occur naturally in the soil as a result of bacterial action which involves capturing nitrogen directly from the air. With the discovery in the 1930s of a way of extracting nitrogen from the atmosphere in large chemical plants, the use of nitrates escalated. As part of fertiliser, nitrates are used to increase grass production which ultimately increases the supply of dairy products and meat. However, a considerable amount of the fertiliser is absorbed into the soil or washed off the surface, particularly by the action of rain, ending up in the food and water supply. This is particularly true for fruit and vegetables that are picked before they are ripe. Although nitrates are used by the plant during the growth or ripening process, they are stored in the tissues beforehand and will remain there if the plant is harvested prematurely. Nitrates, as well as other chemical substances, are known to inhibit enzyme activity, thus potentially affecting body metabolism.

The loss of hedgerows, also exacerbated by modern agricultural practices, causes soil erosion as well as removing the habitat for certain wildlife. Organically farmed fields, on the other hand, are kept small and this allows for the preservation of walls and hedges.

Over 90% of all fruits, vegetables and cereals are sprayed with one or more forms of pesticide. Spraying is often done as a matter of routine rather than only when necessary. Pests become resistant to these agents in a similar way that germs develop resistance to antibiotics. Just as increasing the dose of antibiotics is the typical response, so an increase in the number of times a field is sprayed or more powerful chemicals are employed are the typical actions. We end up with residues from pesticides as part of the 'food' we eat. Pesticides have also been shown to be toxic to wildlife, as one might expect.

There are more than 2500 pesticide products available. A fruit, for example, may be sprayed with as many as 40 different chemicals before it reaches the kitchen. It may have been inflicted with substances designed to do everything from killing insect pests and destroying weeds to assisting the initial growth. There are growth retardants to avoid the growth of excess branches on the parent plant, colour enhancers to speed up ripening, hormones to prevent the fruit from falling naturally from the tree until they are large enough for market, fungicides to prevent rotting . . . and the list goes on.

So what do all these chemicals used in fertilisers and pesticides actually do to human health, and are they really necessary anyway? A brief look at their history is very revealing. In the middle of the last century a German chemist, Justus von Leibig, reasoned that a combination of nitrogen, phosphorus and potash (potassium) were the ingredients that gave nourishment to plants. This soon led to the commercial development of synthetic chemicals. Potassium salts were exported to the United States until the First World War, when native deposits were found, and this launched the manufacture of chemical fertilisers in America.

Prior to von Liebig's 'discovery', humus (organic soil material resulting from partial decomposition of plant and animal matter) was considered to be the primary source of plant nourishment. In fact, 10 years after his 'discovery', von Liebig recognised that he had made a mistake. However, this realisation came too late as profits were already on the rise at the chemical companies. New discoveries in chemistry opened the way for an endless number of compounds to be produced. This enabled companies to continue to bring out new improved varieties, which feeds into the ever-increasing circles caused by pest resistance.

Concern over the effects of fertilisers and pesticides on health and the environment is not new. In 1912 Dr Alexis Carrel, a Nobel Prize winner, felt that the only way to create a healthy world would be to re-establish balance in a soil which had been tampered with due to modern farming methods. He was by no means alone in this belief. Many knowledgeable people were in agreement then, as now, that the real root of malnutrition can be traced back to the soil. It is a fact that good health depends on nutritious food. All food stems from the soil whether it is the fruits, vegetables, nuts and grains that we eat directly or the meat and dairy products provided by animals which are nurtured by these sources. The quality of our food can be no better than the quality of the soil from which it comes. If soil is deficient in trace nutrients, which can be destroyed as a result of chemicals, then it follows that food and indeed water will suffer the same fate.

Sir Albert Howard, an ICI (then Imperial Chemicals) botanist and British colonial officer working in India, was sure that more harm than good was being caused by chemical fertilisers. By 1916, as a result of numerous experiments, he became convinced that these fertilisers, although initially able to stimulate plant growth, were actually destroying the life and vitality of the topsoil. He was also able to prove that livestock fed on organically grown fodder were resistant to disease.

Sir Albert returned to England in the early 1930s, and set about writing up his research. His conclusions, that many of the diseases that are found in plants, animals and humans are a direct result of the use of chemical fertilisers, was met with disdain.

It was Lady Eve Balfour, one of Sir Albert's supporters, who founded The Soil Association in 1946 after receiving a positive response from her book, *The Living Soil*, which had been published in 1943. The aim of the association was to explore the links between soil, plant, animal and man. The practice of organic methods was implemented on an agricultural scale.

In 1955, Lawrence Hills set up the Henry Doubleday Research Association. The aim was to carry out practical research on organic gardening. The association is currently co-ordinating a world-wide programme to establish sustainable farming systems. Hopefully this will help curtail the export of these artificial agricultural methods to the Third World, where some of the problems discussed above are beginning to appear. Outrageously, a number of chemicals that have already been banned in the West are being sold there.

Dr William Rea, who is the Director of The Environmental Health Center in Dallas, Texas, as well as holder of the First World Professional Chair in Environmental Medicine at the Robens Institute, University of Surrey, has concluded that, 'pesticides have the ability to severely disturb the immune system' (see 'Don't Get Sprayed', *Here's Health*, May, 1990). As is clear from the review of modern degenerative diseases described in Chapter 4, a failure of the immune system is in fact the common denominator of many of them.

The practice of organic growing methods can do much to

Table 9: An outline of organic growing methods

The principles of organic growing, which relies more on a knowledge of ecology rather than one of chemistry, include:

crop rotation – builds up soil fertility while destroying the life cycle of crop-specific pests;

natural fertilisers – by recycling nutrients through composting and careful use of animal manure;

non-chemical pest and weed control – chemical pesticides can be dangerous to wildlife (including human health);

minimise the use of fossil fuels in agriculture;

mixed farming – a combination of arable crops and livestock and/or permaculture; crops dependant on each other for things like fertilisation, water, pollination and pest control;

respect for wildlife and the countryside;

humane treatment of farm animals – free access to pastures and no unnecessary drug or hormone treatment.

improve the health of the soil and the plants and animals which depend on it (see Table 9). One example of a natural pesticide is garlic, planted between rows of vegetables which may be specifically vulnerable to insect attacks. Garlic can help protect the plants from insect infestation. Kelp, a common seaweed, is a beneficial fertiliser because it supplies a number of minerals and helps to oxygenate the soil.

A concern to farmers, who may be contemplating returning to a more natural approach to farming, is the conversion time that is necessary to allow the natural system to become re-established. Natural pest predators, which have more than likely been killed off by the pesticides as well, must also be given time to return. It is clear that farmers turning to organic methods will need grant support during this changeover period. At long last, the government has recognised the need for more organic farming, and seems to be taking these difficulties on board, at least to some extent. Big business, too, is getting involved: the managing director of Safeways Supermarket chain has recently called for another 10 000 organic farms. He made the point that the organic vegetables in his shops should be cheaper than the chemically-assisted non-organic equivalent, if the energy costs involved in their production was to be fully compared. Currently, the reverse is true, and organic produce costs more, a situation that can only be put right by greater organic supply.

Against a return to organic farming methods must be placed the alternative: damage to the environment; health hazards due to pesticides in the food chain; overall reduction in food quality; and a depletion of non-renewable resources. No doubt there are a number of other items that may be added to this list.

With some degree of effort on the part of the consumer, organic versions of most food sources including fruits, vegetables, cereals, dairy products, meats and even wine can now be obtained.

We can help to ensure that more stores start stocking these products simply by requesting them to do so — shop managers are becoming increasingly responsive to such customer demand. We must, however, show our support by being willing to spend a little extra for these products. In time, and with more and more people joining in this effort, prices will start to come down.

If we wish, we can strive for and indeed reach the ultimate aim of having truly healthy foods available at prices that match, and perhaps even undercut, those of the nutritionally deficient variety that most of us have been forced to buy due to lack of choice. Surely the nutritional superiority, better taste and contribution to helping clean up the environment that such foods offer make them and us worth it?

A 'DROP' ON WATER

The fact that some of the water that flows through the taps of many houses in Britain is in breach of the Maximum Admissible Concentration levels of toxins set by the EC in 1980 should be an outrage to every citizen. These concentrations can be made up of lead, aluminium, nitrates, pesticides and other potentially harmful substances. As discussed above, nitrates from fertilisers, and probably pesticides as well, can wash off the land surface or percolate through the upper layers of soil ending up in nearby water courses. High levels of nitrates can lead to a lowering of oxygen levels in lakes, rivers and streams thus affecting aquatic life (and, ultimately, the oceans).

Many people now buy bottled water to use for drinking, and some have filters to help eliminate some of these elements from their water supply. We pay for the water that we receive, are we not entitled to a say in its quality?.

WHAT CAN WE DO?

In summary, then, here are a few pointers to assist the development of the health and ecological aspects of diet.

• buy local produce from local shops. This helps to eliminate excess packaging and energy used in transport;
• buy meat, milk or eggs that comes only from free range-fed animals, preferably those fed only on organic feed;
• try using soya milk as a dairy milk substitute;
• insist on organic vegetables, fruits and grains. When not available, choose fruit and vegetables that are in season as they may not be as heavily chemically treated.

If these matters are of concern to you, write to your local MP demanding:

• adequate government grants and subsidies for organic farming;
• a national pesticide policy that takes into account all aspects of a complicated issue, including those of the consumer;
• that schools be provided with teaching aids from such groups as The Soil Association (and others listed in the reference section — see Useful addresses).

Finally, do what you can to recycle as many things as possible. Most towns now have bottle banks and paper depositories. Other recyclables include aluminium cans, plastic bags, and organic waste from food sources which can be turned into compost. Even old wellies are being recycled in some countries! Keep informed by joining an environment group — see Useful addresses.

Keep in the forefront of your mind that, collectively, we possess the power to change any situation . . . and that time is running out.

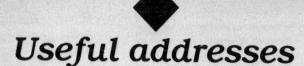

Useful addresses

NOTE: When requesting information remember to include an SAE.

ORGANISATIONS CONCERNED WITH SPECIFIC DISEASES

ME Action Campaign, PO Box 1126, London W3 0RY.

ARMS (Action for Research into Multiple Sclerosis), 4A Chapel Hill, Stansted, Essex CM24 8AG. Tel: 0279 815553.

Bristol Cancer Help Centre, Grove House, Cornwallis Grove, Clifton, Bristol BS8 4PG. Tel: 0272 743216.

New Approaches to Cancer, 5 Larksfield, Egham, Surrey TW20 0RB. Tel: 0784 433610.
> An umbrella organisation for about 300 groups throughout the UK with overseas contacts as well.

Springhill Centre, Cuddington Road, Dinton, Nr. Aylesbury, Bucks HP18 0AD. Tel: 0296 748278.
> A charity entirely dedicated to the welfare of the severely ill, their families and friends. Offers a holistic approach to caring, and healing of life-threatening diseases in both their Day Care Centre and Residential Hospice.

Gerson Institute, PO Box 430, Bonita, California, 92002, USA.

Action Against Allergy, Greyhound House, 23/24 George Street, Richmond, Surrey TW9 1JY.

The British Diabetic Association, 10 Queen Anne Street, London W1M 0BD. Tel: 071-323 1531.

National Eczema Society, Tavistock House North, Tavistock Square, London WC1H 9SR. Tel: 071-388 4097.

Environment for Hypersensitives Organisation, 5 Kilham, Orton Goldhay, Peterborough, Cambs PE2 0SU.

British Association of Cancer United Patients (BACUP), 121/123 Charterhouse Street, London EC1M 6AA. Tel: in London 071-608 1661 or outside London Freeline 0800 181199.
Provides information, advice and support to cancer patients, their families and friends.

The British Nutrition Foundation, 15 Belgrave Square, London SW1X 8PG. (Booklet 'Eating for a Healthier Heart').

ECOLOGY

The Soil Association, 86-88 Colston Street, Bristol BS1.
Supplies a list of organic meat suppliers and information on courses in organic farming and gardening in the United Kingdom.

Henry Doubleday Research Association, National Centre for Organic Gardening, Ryton on Dunsmore, Coventry CV8 3LG. Tel: 0203 303517.
Information on courses in organic gardening and farming in the United Kingdom.

Elm Farm Research Centre, Hamstead Marshall, Nr Newbury, Berkshire RG15 0HR. Tel: 0488 58298.
An organic mixed farm where new developments in methods and techniques are researched and demonstrated – research papers, booklets and soil analysis service are available.

Working Weekends on Organic Farms (WWOOF), 19 Bradford Road, Lewes, Sussex BN7 1RB. (Contact is by post, they request that no one comes without an appointment.)

Living Earth Ltd, 10 Upper Grosvenor Street, London W1X 9PA. Tel: 071-499 0854.

> Works with schools and local communities to provide environmental education, information, expertise and practical help.

Organic Growers Association, 86 Colston Street, Bristol BS1 5BB. Tel: 0272 299800/299666.

Organic Farming Centre, The Edinburgh School of Agriculture, West Mains Road, Edinburgh EH9 3JG. Tel: 031-667 6914.

The Permaculture Association, 8 Hunters Moon, Dartington, Totnes, Devon TQ9 6JT. Tel: 0803 865115.

Green Farm Nutrition Centre, Burwash Common, East Sussex TN19 7LX.

> Information available for growing your own organic vegetables and herbs.

Earth Resources Research Ltd, 258 Pentonville Road, London N1 9JY. Tel: 071-278 3833.

Friends of the Earth, 26-28 Underwood Street, London N1. Tel: 071-490 1555.

Pesticides Trust, 20 Compton Terrace, London N1 2VN. Tel: 071-354 3860.

Pesticide Exposure Group Sufferers, c/o Enfys Chapman, 10 Parker Street, Cambridge.

> Helps victims pursue compensation claims (Enfys Chapman founded the group after being a victim herself – she is presently confined to a wheelchair).

ANIMAL RIGHTS

Animal Aid, 7 Castle Street, Tonbridge, Kent TN9 1BH. (If requesting information to be sent do send a SAE and if you can afford it a small donation.)

Compassion in World Farming, 20 Lavant Street, Petersfield, Hampshire GU32 3EW. Tel: 0730 64208/68863.

The Free Range Egg Association, 37 Tanza Road, London NW3 2UA. (Supplies a list of free range egg producers.)

The Real Meat Company Ltd, East Hill Farm, Heystesbury, Warminster, Wilts, BA12 0HR. (Supplies a list of humane meat suppliers.)

OTHER USEFUL ADDRESSES

The London Food Commission, 88 Old Street, London EC1V 9AR.

Institute of Complementary Medicine, 21 Portland Place, London W1.

Parents for Safe Food, Britannia House, 1/11 Glenthorne Road, London W1. Tel: 071-748 9898, ext. 330.
Also campaigns for greater awareness of the potential exposure to pesticides.

Institute of Optimum Nutrition, 8 Jerdan Place, London SW6 1BE.

Food Watch International, Butts Pond Industrial Estate, Sturminster Newton, Dorset DT10 1AZ. Tel: 0258 73356.
Supplies food, on a mail order basis, for people intolerant to various ingredients and additives.

Colonic International Association, 26a Sea Road, Boscombe, Bournemouth, Dorset BH5 1DF.

Green Farm Nutrition Centre, Burwash Common, East Sussex TN19 7IX.

Glossary of terms

Alimentary canal: the long passage, extending from the mouth to the anus, through which food passes to be digested and absorbed.

Amino acids: fundamental constituents of all proteins. There are 22 different amino acids, of which the body can synthesise all but nine. These nine must be obtained from food sources.

Antibody: special blood protein produced by the body to control any substance introduced into the body which is considered dangerous.

Antigen: any substance, such as a virus, considered dangerous by the body and against which it produces a specific antibody.

Antioxidant: a substance that protects food from oxidation. Nutrients that act as antioxidants include vitamins C and E, beta-carotene and selenium.

Calorie: a unit of energy which is provided by an item of food. The calorie content of a food is determined by the rise in temperature of the food source when it is heated (a measurement of the energy released).

Cardiovascular: consisting of the heart and two networks of blood vessels which together effect the circulation of blood throughout the body.

Co-enzyme: a non-protein organic compound that, in the presence of an enzyme, plays an essential role in the reaction that is catalysed by the enzyme.

Complex carbohydrate: a substance made up of the elements carbon, hydrogen and oxygen, usually referred to as a starch, and together with micronutrients, water and fibre forming a complex that is characteristic for each plant.

DNA (deoxyribonucleic acid): genetic material of nearly all living organisms which controls heredity and is located in the nucleus of cells.

Duodenum: the first section of the three-part small intestines.

Enzyme: a protein catalyst. In small amounts, speeds up the rate of a biological reaction without itself being used up in the reaction.

Free radicals: produced from many outside sources such as X-rays and the heating of vegetable oils, as well as from the body itself; these substances can attach themselves to other substances in the body causing damage to cell membranes and DNA structures which can lead to cancerous mutations.

Glucose: a simple sugar and important source of energy in the body and the sole source of energy for the brain.

Gluten: an elastic protein substance which is found in wheat and rye. Gluten becomes sticky when wet and converts elasticity to dough.

Glycoprotein: one of a group of compounds consisting of protein combined with a carbohydrate – usually part of enzymes, hormones or antigens.

Hormones: internal secretions produced by ductless glands in the body that travel via the bloodstream to other parts of the body to help modify function or structure.

Histidine: an essential amino acid needed primarily by children; involved in the growth process.

Hyperglycaemia: excess of glucose in the bloodstream.

Can be caused by insufficient insulin in the blood and excessive intake of carbohydrates.

Hypoglycaemia: deficiency of glucose in the bloodstream causing muscular weakness, mental confusion and sweating. Can occur as a result of insulin overdose in diabetics.

Iatrogenic: a condition that results from treatment. It can be either an inevitable or unforeseen side-effect.

Isoleucine: an essential amino acid.

Leucine: an essential amino acid.

Linolenic acid: an essential fatty acid.

Lysine: an essential amino acid.

Methionine: an essential amino acid used to make keratin, found in insulin and hair.

Myelin: formed from protein, myelin is laid down as a sheath around certain nerve fibres, allowing these nerves to conduct impulses more rapidly.

Nucleic acids: either of two organic acids, DNA or RNA, present in the nucleus of all living cells. Their main functions are in heredity and protein synthesis.

Omega 3, 6, or 9: the three categories of unsaturated fats. The difference is determined by where the first double bond on the fatty acid chain occurs.

Peristalsis: involuntary wavelike movement that progresses along some of the hollow tubes of the body such as the gut.

Permaculture: growing many crops which regulate one another and need little or no maintenance.

Pesticide (chemical): poisons which are designed to kill insects, weeds, fungi, moulds, rats and other 'pest' species.

Phenylalanine: an essential amino acid.

Prostaglandin: one of a group of hormone-like substances present in a wide variety of tissues and body fluids.

RNA (ribonucleic acid): concerned with the synthesis of proteins and found in the nucleus of cells.

Sebum: thin film of fat, secreted by glands, which spreads over the skin and slows the evaporation of water; also has an antibacterial effect.

Soya bean: a legume known as 'the cow of the orient'.

Sucrose: human-refined sugar and the principal constituent of cane sugar and sugar beet. A carbohydrate consisting of glucose and fructose.

Threonine: an essential amino acid.

Tocopherol: name first given to what is now commonly known as vitamin E. The word literally means the ability to reproduce.

Toxicity: the quality or condition of being poisonous or destructive.

Tryptophan: an essential amino acid.

Typhoid: infection of the digestive system caused by the bacterium *Salmonella typhi.* Transmitted through contaminated food and drink.

Typhus: infection caused by a particular parasitic organism that is transmitted to man via lice or mites.

Valine: an essential amino acid.

Yellow fever: infectious disease caused by a virus transmitted to man by mosquitoes. The virus causes degeneration of the liver and kidneys.

▶ GO TO ▶   ◆ *Healthy foods — where to find them, page 187*
◆ *Food ecology, page 217*

Bibliography

CHAPTER 1: BEING OVERWEIGHT

Adams, Gill. 'Eating for a Good Life', *Family Circle*, July, 1990.

Angier, Natalie. 'Fat on Thighs and Paunches is the Fate of all Mammals', *The New York Times*, October 30, 1990.

Cobb, Dr John. 'I Feel So Guilty', *Slimming Magazine*, 1990.

Cobb, Dr John. 'Slim Success – What Should You do if it Scares you?', *Slimming Magazine*, 1990.

Cobb, Dr John. 'Stress, Nine Ways to Save Yourself', *Slimming Magazine*, 1990.

Colleee, John. 'A Doctor Writes', *The Observer*, 1990.

Fredericks, Carlton PhD. *Psycho-Nutrition*, Grosset & Dunlap, New York, 1976.

Graf, Eva and Jordan, Mary Kate. *Choices: How to Win Your Fight with the Dragon*, Center of the Light, 1981.

Katz, Richard. *Boiling Energy*, Harvard University Press, 1982.

Kent, Ann. 'Can Your Mind Really Affect your Health?'', *Practical Heath*, 1990.

Look After Yourself! Health Guide, The Health Education Council.

McLaughlin, Chris. 'Depression: There is a Positive Approach', *Practical Health*, 1990.

Murray, Michael and Pizorno, Joseph. *Encyclopaedia of Natural Medicine*, Optima, 1990.

Robinson, Corinne H. and Lawler, Marilyn, R. *Normal and Therapeutic Nutrition*, Macmillan, New York, 1982.

Tarnower, Dr H. *The Complete Scarsdale Diet*, Bantam Books, 1980.

CHAPTER 2: BEING UNDERWEIGHT

Null, Gary and Null, Steven. *How to Get Rid of the Poisons in Your Body*, Arco Publishing, New York, 1984.

Phillips, Phoebe and Hatch, Pamela (Eds). *The Best of Good Health*, Book Club Associates, London, 1978.

CHAPTER 3: WHY 'ORDINARY' DIETS DO NOT WORK

Black, Maggie. *Food and Cooking in Medieval Britain*, English Heritage, 1985.

Dufty, William. *Sugar Blues*, Chilton Book Company, Pennsylvania, USA, 1975.

Mottram, Professor V. H. *Food Sense*, Ward Lock, 1953.

CHAPTER 4: A–Z OF DIET-RELATED DISEASE

Adams, F. *The Genuine Works of Hippocrates*, Williams & Williams, Baltimore, Maryland, 1939.

Airola, Paavo PhD. *The Miracle of Garlic*, Health Plus Publishers, Arizona, USA, 1978.

All About the Irritable Bowel Syndrome, The British Digestive Foundation.

All About Ulcers, The British Digestive Foundation.

Allergy and Food Intolerance Factsheet, ME Action Campaign.

Archer, Anne. 'A Cancer Therapy that Refuses to be Ignored', *Journal of Alternative Medicine*, October, 1985.

Becker, Robert O. MD. *Cross Currents*, Jeremy P. Tarcher Inc., 1990.

'Bristol Study Team Admits Getting it Wrong', *Here's Health*, January 1991.

Chaitow, Leon. *Arthritis Self Help*, Thorsons, 1987.

Chaitow, Leon. *Candida Albicans – Could Yeast be Your Problem?*, Thorsons, 1985.

Clyne, Rachael. *Coping with Cancer*, Thorsons, 1986.

Coleman, Pearl. 'Helping to Beat the Candida Scourge', *Journal of Alternative Medicine*, August, 1985.

Cooke, A.M. (Ed.). *The Royal Society of Medicine Family Medical Guide*, (1980), Perrage Books, 1988.

Crook, William G. MD. *The Yeast Connection*, Professional Books, 1983.

De Vries, Jan. *Body Energy*, Mainstream Publishing, 1989.

Diet Factsheet, ME Action Campaign.

Eaton, S.B., Shostak, M. and Konner, M. *The Stone-Age Health Programme*, Angus & Robertson, 1988.

Edwards, David and Bazalgette, Peter. *BBC Food Check*, BBC Books, 1989.

Evans, John. 'New Theory of Cancer', *Journal of Alternative and Complementary Medicine*, March 1989.

Fredericks, Carlton PhD. *Psycho-Nutrition*, Grosset & Dunlap, New York, 1976.

Gerson, Max MD. *A Cancer Therapy*, Gerson Institute, California, 1986.

Govindji, Azmina. 'Diabetic Foods – Do We Need Them?', *Balance*, April/May 1989.

Haught, S.J. *Cancer? Think Curable!*, Gerson Institute, California, 1983.

Heinerman, John. *Science of Herbal Medicine*, Bi-World Publishers, 1979.

Introducing Diabetes, British Diabetic Association, January 1988.

Jacobs, Gill. *Candida Albicans*, Optima, 1990.

Kenton, Leslie; Kenton, Susannah. *Raw Energy*, Arrow Books, 1989.

Kidman, Brenda. *A Gentle Way with Cancer*, Century Arrow, 1986.

Kowalski, Robert E. *The 8-Week Cholesterol Cure*, Thorsons, 1990.

Lamont, Keith. 'Check your Reaction to Hypoglycaemia', *Journal of Alternative Medicine*, 1985.

LeShan, Lawrence PhD. *Cancer as a Turning Point*, Gateway Books, 1990.

Leung, A.Y. *Encyclopaedia of Common Natural Ingredients used in Foods, Drugs and Cosmetics*, John Wiley, New York, 1980.

Lust, John. *The Herb Book*, Bantam Books, 1974.

Mackarness, Dr Richard. *Not all in the Mind*, Pan Books, 1976.

Mayes, Kathleen, *Brittle Bones and the Calcium Crisis*, Thorsons, 1987.

Miller, Jonathan D. *Candida Yeast – the Battle in your Body*, Life Circle, Ohio, 1986.

Moore Lappé, Frances. *Diet for a Small Planet*, Ballantine Books, 1982.

National Eczema Society – Diet and Children with Eczema, National Eczema Society, 1986.

Null, Gary. 'Cancer Part II: Alternative Therapies', *Natural Living Newsletter,* Vol. 1, No. 8.

Null, Gary. 'Cancer Part III: Alternative Therapies', *Natural Living Newsletter,* Vol. 2, No. 1.

Null, Gary. 'Why we are Losing the War on Cancer', *Natural Living Newsletter,* Vol. 1, No.4.

Null, Gary. 'Candida (Yeast Infections)', *Natural Living Newsletter,* No. 29

Robbins, John. *Diet for a New America,* Stillpoint, USA, 1987.

Shallis, Michael. *The Electric Shock Book,* Souvenir Press, 1988.

Shreeve, Dr Caroline. 'Cancer and Natural Nutrients', *The Vitamin Connection,* Jan/Feb 1990.

Shreeve, Dr Caroline M. *Lower Your Blood Pressure in 4 Easy Stages,* Thorsons, 1989.

Simpson, H.C.R., Lousley, S., Geekie, M., *et al.* 'A High Carbohydrate Leguminous Fibre Diet Improves all Aspects of Diabetic Control', *Lancet,* 3 January, 1981.

Stanway, Penny. *Diet for Common Ailments,* Sidgwick & Jackson, 1989.

Thorson's Editorial Board, *The Complete Raw Juice Therapy,* Thorsons, 1989.

Wachman, Amnon and Berstein, Daniel S. 'Diet and Osteoporosis', *Lancet,* May, 1968.

Williams, Roger J. *Nutrition Against Disease,* Bantam Books, 1981.

CHAPTER 5: GRADUAL WEIGHT LOSS TECHNIQUES

Webb, Lizzie. 'The Dangers of Exercise', *Slimming Magazine*, 1990.

CHAPTER 6: QUICK WEIGHT LOSS TECHNIQUES

Marsden, Kathryn. 'Nutritional Counselling', *Healthy Eating*, Feb/March, 1990.

CHAPTER 7: GUIDELINES FOR CREATING A HEALTHY DIET

Burl, Aubrey. *Prehistoric Avebury*, Yale University Press, 1979.

Diet and Nutrition, Superdrug, Octopus Books, 1985.

Ehmke, J. Ehmke, K. and Krantz, Larry. *Food for Life*, Whole Health Institute, USA, 1989.

Holford, Patrick. 'Nutrition: Holford's Hints', *Journal of Alternative & Complementary Medicine*, March, 1989.

Martin, Sara. 'A Process of Elimination', *Here's Health*, March, 1988.

Melville, Arabella and Johnson, Colin. *Persistent Fat and How to Lose it*, Guild Publishing, 1986.

Pritikin, Nathan. *Pritikin Program for Diet & Exercise*, Bantam Books, 1990.

Proposed Nutritional Guidelines for a Healthier Diet Made Simple, Safeway Nutritional Advice Service.

CHAPTER 8: SUBSTITUTING HEALTHY FOR LESS HEALTHY FOODS

Diet and Nutrition, Superdrug, Octopus Books, 1985.

Ehmke, J., Ehmke, K. and Krantz, Larry. *Food for Life*, Whole Health Institute, USA, 1989.

Holford, Patrick. 'Nutrition: Holford's Hints', *Journal of Alternative & Complementary Medicine*, March, 1989.

Pritikin, Nathan. *Pritikin Program for Diet & Exercise*, Bantam Books, 1990.

Proposed Nutritional Guidelines for a Healthier Diet Made Simple, Safeway Nutritional Advice Service.

CHAPTER 9: MAINTAINING HEALTHY WEIGHT GAIN

Pyke, Magnus. *Success in Nutrition*, John Murray, 1975.

CHAPTER 10: MAINTAINING HEALTHY WEIGHT LOSS

Erdmann, Robert PhD. and Jones, Meirion. *Fats, Nutrition and Health*, Thorsons, 1990.

'The Hunger Control Diet', *Slimming Magazine*, 1990.

'Your Greatest Guide to Calories', *Slimming Magazine*, February 1990.

CHAPTER 11: COMMON SENSE TIPS FOR KEEPING TO A DIET

'Fast Foods – Too Much for our Children to Swallow?', *Practical Health*, 1990.

Mulherin, Jennifer. *Spices and Natural Flavourings*, Ward Lock, 1988.

Stuart, Malcolm (Ed.). *The Encyclopaedia of Herbs and Herbalism*, Crescent Books, New York, 1979.

Trewby, Mary. *A Gourmet's Book of Herbs & Spices*, Salamander Books, 1989.

CHAPTER 12: A-Z OF DIETS TO COMBAT DISEASE

Golos, N. and Golos F.G. *Coping with your Allergies*, Simon & Schuster, New York, 1986.

Randolph, T.G. and Moss, R.W. *An Alternative Approach to Allergies*, Bantam Books, New York, 1980.

Shreeve, Dr Caroline. 'Dietary Help for Thrush', *Healthy Eating*, Feb/March 1990.

CHAPTER 13: WEIGHT LOSS GROUPS AND 'WONDER' DIETS

Conley, Rosemary. *Hip and Thigh Diet*, Arrow, 1989.

Jarvis, D.C. MD. *Folk Medicine*, Pan Books, 1975.

Mazel, Judy. *The Beverly Hills Diet*, Sidgwick & Jackson, 1982.

CHAPTER 14: GUIDE TO NUTRIENTS, VITAMINS AND MINERALS

Cameron, Ewan and Pauling, Linus. *Cancer and Vitamin C*, Warner Books, New York, 1981.

Chaitow, Leon. *Arthritis*, Thorsons, 1987.

Chaitow, Leon. *Clear Body, Clear Mind*, Unwin Hyman, 1990.

Chaitow, Leon. 'Vitamin A: All the Practitioner Need Know', *Journal of Alternative Medicine*, June, 1983.

NUTRITION AND DIET LOGIC

'Cholesterol How Much is Too Much', *The Vitamin Connection*, Nov/Dec, 1988.

'Eating for a Healthier Heart', *British Nutrition Foundation*.

Fat, Safeway Healthy Living Guide No. 7.

Hill, Ray. 'Let's Explain the For's and Against's the Fats and Oils', *Health Guardian*, 1990.

Holland & Barrett Vitamins and Minerals, Thorsons, 1986.

Holmes, Valerie. 'Vitamin E: A Changing View', *Healthy Eating*, Feb/March, 1990.

'The Many Faces of Zinc', *The Vitamin Connection*, Nov/Dec, 1988.

Mervyn, L. *The Dictionary of Minerals*, Thorsons, 1985.

Mervyn, L. *The B Vitamins*, Thorsons, 1981.

Mindell, Earl L. 'Trace Minerals and Immunity', *The Vitamin Connection*, Nov/Dec, 1988.

Mindell, Earl. 'Does Nutrition Affect the Health of Your Skin and Hair', *Healthy Eating*, Feb/March 1990.

Mott, Auriel. 'Sounds Fishy', *The Vitamin Connection*, Jan/Feb 1990.

Null, Gary. 'Calcium', *Natural Living Newsletter*, No. 12.

Null, Gary. 'Vitamin A', *Natural Living Newsletter*, No. 17.

Null, Gary. 'Vitamin B Complex: Part I' and 'Part II', *Natural Living Newsletters*, Nos. 25 & 26.

Null, Gary. 'Vitamin C', *Natural Living Newsletter*, No. 18.

Null, Gary. 'Vitamin E', *Natural Living Newsletter*, No. 21.

Rivers, John. 'The Vitamin Collection', *The Vitamin Connection*, Nov/Dec, 1988.

'Selenium Synergy the Key to Disease Protection', *Journal of Alternative Medicine*, May, 1985.

Smith, Angela, 'Natural Protection' and 'Minerally Speaking', *The Vitamin Connection*, Jan/Feb, 1990.

Stanway, Dr Andrew. *Trace Elements*, Van Dyke Books, 1983.

Stone, Irwin. *The Healing Factor: Vitamin C Against Disease*, Grosset & Dunlap, New York, 1972.

'An Update on Beta Carotene', *The Vitamin Connection*, Jan/Feb 1990.

CHAPTER 15: VEGETARIAN AND OTHER ALTERNATIVE DIETS

Cook, John. *Diet and Your Religion*, Woodbridge Press, Santa Barbara, California, 1976.

Leung, Albert. *Chinese Herbal Remedies*, Universe Books, New York, 1984.

Sweet, Amanda. *The Vegan Health Plan*, Arlington Books, 1987.

Walker, Dr Morton. 'The Japanese Diet', *Healthy Eating*, Feb/March 1990.

CHAPTER 16: HEALTHY ALTERNATIVE FOODS AND WHERE TO FIND THEM

Chaitow, Leon and Trenev, Natasha. 'Yoghurt Healthfood or Health Fraud?', *Here's Health*, March 1990.

Culpeper's Complete Herbal & English Physician, Pitman Press Ltd, 1981 (reproduced from an original edition published in 1826).

NUTRITION AND DIET LOGIC

'Easy Meals – Quorn', *Journal of Complementary Medicine*, March 1989.

Fulder, Dr Stephen. 'The Magic of Garlic', *Health Guardian.*

Goulart, Frances S. *The Carob Way to Health*, Warner Books, USA, 1982.

Hagler, Louise. *Tofu Cookery*, The Book Publishing Company, USA, 1982.

Leng, Vikki. *Vegetarian Super Soya Foods*, Thorsons, 1988.

Mabey, Richard. *Food for Free*, Peerage Books, 1986.

MacNeil, Karen. *The Book of Whole Foods*, Robert Hale, 1986.

Mulkern, Becky. *The Healing Properties of Garlic*, Earth Star Press.

Null, Gary. *The New Vegetarian Cookbook*, Collier Mac-Millan, 1980.

Oliver, Martha H. *Add a Few Sprouts*, Keats Publishing Co., 1975.

Powell, Eric F.W. *Kelp the Health Giver*, Health Science Press, 1980.

'Quorn Press Release Kit', Wearne Public Relations, London.

Roser, David. 'Garlic is Good for You – Official!', *Healthy Eating*, Feb/March 1990.

Shurtleff, William and Auyagi, Akiko. *The Book of Tofu*, Ballantine, 1975.

Spencer, Colin. 'A Protein Plant for the Palate', *Weekend Guardian*, 1 & 2 December, 1990.

Stein, Irene. *Royal Jelly*, Thorsons, 1986.

Zen Cookery, Practical Macrobiotics, The Ohsawa Foundation, Los Angeles, California.

CHAPTER 17: FOOD SAFETY

Additives: Why do we Need Them?, Safeway Nutrition Advice Service.

Chance, Susie. 'Honey: How Sweet It Is', *Healthy Eating*, Feb/March 1990.

Food Additives — the Balanced Approach, Ministry of Agriculture, Fisheries and Food, 1987.

Hanssen, Maurice. *The New E for Additives*, Thorsons, 1987.

Kenton, Leslie and Kenton, Susannah. *Raw Energy Recipes*, Century Publishing, 1985.

Laurent, Claire. 'Food Irradiation The Whole Story', *Practical Health*, 1990.

Look at the Label, Ministry of Agriculture, Fisheries and Food, 1988.

Mellis, Sue and Davidson, Barbara. *The Born-Again Carnivore*, Optima, 1990.

Mott, Auriel. 'In Food We Trust', *The Vitamin Connection*, Jan/Feb 1990.

Piccioni, Richard. 'Food Irradiation: Contaminating our Food', *The Ecologist*, Vol. 18, Nos. 2 & 3, 1988.

Smith, Jill. 'Suffering of Salmon', *Resurgence*, Sept/Oct 1989.

Spencer, Colin. 'Irradiation? No Thanks', *Weekend Guardian*, 3-4 February 1990.

Webb, Tony and Lang, Tim. *Food Irradiation, The Myth and the Reality*, Thorsons, 1990.

CHAPTER 18: FOOD ECOLOGY

'Deadly Cow Brain Disease Fears Increase', *Agscene*, No. 98, Spring 1990.

Epstein, Samuel S. MD. 'BST: The Public Health Hazards', *The Ecologist*, Vol. 19, No. 5, Sept/Oct 1989.

Fact Sheet – Eating the Cruelty-Free Way, Compassion in World Farming.

Factory Farming Today, Compassion in World Farming.

Ferriman, Annabel and Ghazi, Polly. 'The Rot in John Bull's Beef', *Sunday Observer, 20 May 1990.*

Glew, Jenny. *'Practically Green', Practical Health,* 1990.

Loads More Muck and Magic, Channel 4 Television, 1990.

Mabey, D. Gear, A. and Gear, J. (Eds). *Organic Consumer Guide*, Thorsons, 1990.

McKinley, Philippa. 'Don't Get Sprayed', *Here's Health*, May 1990.

Milked for all She's Worth, Compassion in World Farming.

Mott, Auriel. 'Holding Water', *Healthy Eating*, Feb/March 1990.

Tompkins, Peter and Bird, Christopher. *Secrets of the Soil*, Harper & Row, 1989.

Tyler, Andrew. 'Pigs Diary', *Animal Aid.*

Tyler, Andrew. 'Don't Look Now, an Everyday Story of Pig Slaughter', *Animal Aid.*

Index